Executive Skills in Children and Adolescents

The Guilford Practical Intervention in the Schools Series
Kenneth W. Merrell, Series Editor

This series presents the most reader-friendly resources available in key areas of evidence-based practice in school settings. Practitioners will find trustworthy guides on effective behavioral, mental health, and academic interventions, and assessment and measurement approaches. Covering all aspects of planning, implementing, and evaluating high-quality services for students, books in the series are carefully crafted for everyday utility. Features include ready-to-use reproducibles, lay-flat binding to facilitate photocopying, appealing visual elements, and an oversized format.

Recent Volumes

School-Based Behavioral Assessment: Informing Intervention and Instruction
Sandra Chafouleas, T. Chris Riley-Tillman, and George Sugai

Collaborating with Parents for Early School Success: The Achieving–Behaving–Caring Program
Stephanie H. McConaughy, Pam Kay, Julie A. Welkowitz, Kim Hewitt, and Martha D. Fitzgerald

Helping Students Overcome Depression and Anxiety, Second Edition: A Practical Guide
Kenneth W. Merrell

Inclusive Assessment and Accountability:
A Guide to Accommodations for Students with Diverse Needs
Sara E. Bolt and Andrew T. Roach

Bullying Prevention and Intervention: Realistic Strategies for Schools
Susan M. Swearer, Dorothy L. Espelage, and Scott A. Napolitano

Conducting School-Based Functional Behavioral Assessments, Second Edition:
A Practitioner's Guide
Mark W. Steege and T. Steuart Watson

Evaluating Educational Interventions:
Single-Case Design for Measuring Response to Intervention
T. Chris Riley-Tillman and Matthew K. Burns

Collaborative Home/School Interventions:
Evidence-Based Solutions for Emotional, Behavioral, and Academic Problems
Gretchen Gimpel Peacock and Brent R. Collett

Social and Emotional Learning in the Classroom:
Promoting Mental Health and Academic Success
Kenneth W. Merrell and Barbara A. Gueldner

Executive Skills in Children and Adolescents, Second Edition:
A Practical Guide to Assessment and Intervention
Peg Dawson and Richard Guare

Responding to Problem Behavior in Schools, Second Edition: The Behavior Education Program
Deanne A. Crone, Leanne S. Hawken, and Robert H. Horner

High-Functioning Autism/Asperger Syndrome in Schools:
Assessment and Intervention
Frank J. Sansosti, Kelly A. Powell-Smith, and Richard J. Cowan

School Discipline and Self-Discipline:
A Practical Guide to Promoting Prosocial Student Behavior
George G. Bear

Executive Skills in Children and Adolescents

A Practical Guide to Assessment and Intervention

SECOND EDITION

PEG DAWSON
RICHARD GUARE

THE GUILFORD PRESS
New York   London

© 2010 The Guilford Press
A Division of Guilford Publications, Inc.
370 Seventh Avenue, Suite 1200, New York, NY 10001
www.guilford.com

Printed in Canada

This book is printed on acid-free paper.

Last digit is print number: 9   8   7   6

Library of Congress Cataloging-in-Publication Data

Dawson, Peg.
    Executive skills in children and adolescents : a practical guide to assessment and intervention /
Peg Dawson and Richard Guare. — 2nd ed.
        p. cm. — (The Guilford practical intervention in the schools series)
    Includes bibliographical references and index.
    ISBN 978-1-60623-571-3 (pbk.: alk. paper)
    1. Executive ability in children.   2. Executive ability in adolescence.   3. Self-management
(Psychology) for teenagers.   4. Self-management (Psychology) for children.   I. Guare, Richard.
II. Title.
    BF723.E93D39 2010
    155.4′13—dc22

                                                                              2009049722

About the Authors

Peg Dawson, EdD, is a staff psychologist at the Center for Learning and Attention Disorders at Seacoast Mental Health Center in Portsmouth, New Hampshire, where she specializes in the assessment of children and adults with learning and attention disorders. She received her doctorate in school/child clinical psychology from the University of Virginia and has worked as a school psychologist in Maine and New Hampshire. Dr. Dawson has many years of organizational experience at the state, national, and international level and has served in many capacities, including President, of the New Hampshire Association of School Psychologists, the National Association of School Psychologists (NASP), and the International School Psychology Association. She is the 2006 recipient of NASP's Lifetime Achievement Award. Dr. Dawson and her colleague Richard Guare have written a manual on coaching students with attention disorders and are the authors of *Smart but Scattered: The Revolutionary "Executive Skills" Approach to Helping Kids Reach Their Potential*, a book for parents on helping children develop executive skills.

Richard Guare, PhD, is a neuropsychologist and board-certified behavior analyst who serves as director of the Center for Learning and Attention Disorders at Seacoast Mental Health Center. He received his doctorate in school/child clinical psychology from the University of Virginia and completed a postdoctoral fellowship in neuropsychology at Children's Hospital Boston. Dr. Guare serves as a consultant to schools and agencies in programs for autism, learning and behavior disorders, and acquired brain injuries. He has presented and published research and clinical work involving attention, executive skills, and neurological disorders. Dr. Guare is coauthor with Peg Dawson of the book *Smart but Scattered* and of a manual on coaching students with attention disorders. He is also coauthor, with Chuck Martin and Peg Dawson, of two books on executive skills of adults in business settings.

Drs. Dawson and Guare's website is *www.smartbutscatteredkids.com.*

Preface

When we published the first edition of *Executive Skills in Children and Adolescents* in 2004, *executive skills* was a relatively new and unfamiliar concept to school psychologists and educators. In the intervening years, the research base has expanded beyond a focus on populations with impairments, such as head injury, to address typical brain development, and the term has become more familiar to parents and teachers alike as they work to understand why some children struggle in school in the absence of an obvious learning disability or emotional disorder. Furthermore, the way schools provide services to students with learning impairments has shifted from a "discrepancy model" to a response-to-intervention (RTI) model along with an emphasis on evidence-based practice. These changes in the field have created a need for a revised and expanded edition of our book.

Executive function is a neuropsychological concept referring to the high-level cognitive processes required to plan and direct activities, including task initiation and follow-through, working memory, sustained attention, performance monitoring, inhibition of impulses, and goal-directed persistence. While the groundwork for development of these executive skills starts before birth, they develop gradually and in a clear progression through the first two decades of life. From the moment that children begin to interact with their environment, adults have expectations for how they will use executive skills to negotiate many of the demands of childhood—from the self-regulation of behavior required to act responsibly to the planning and initiation skills required to complete chores and homework. Parents and teachers expect children to use executive skills even though they may understand little about what these skills are and how they impact behavior and school performance.

Our first encounter with executive skills came through our work with children and teenagers who had sustained traumatic brain injuries. Problems involving planning and organization, time management, and memory, as well as weaknesses with inhibition and regulation of emotions, have long described a significant component of traumatic brain injury. Executive skills have also assumed an increasingly important role in the explanation of attention-deficit/hyperactivity disorder (ADHD). While we were introduced to these skills originally in our work with these populations, we have seen an increasing number of youngsters who seem to struggle in school because of weaknesses in executive skills even when they do not meet the diagnostic criteria for ADHD or another disorder. We believe that these students will benefit from interventions designed to improve executive functioning. To do so, however, requires an understanding of what executive skills are, how they develop in children, and how they impact school performance. This book is intended to shed light on these important cognitive processes so that parents and teachers can better help children hone these skills for the purpose of achieving long-term independence—the ultimate desirable outcome of childhood.

Following the publication of the first edition of this book, we heard from school psychologists and special educators, who found the book invaluable for their daily practice. We also heard from clinical psychologists, neuropsychologists, and pediatric specialists from the medical profession that the book was a useful tool for them in their daily work with children whose problems ranged from the relatively mild issues associated with normal growth and development to the more severe impairments associated with acquired brain injuries, neurological disorders, autism, and ADHD. And, finally, we heard from enough parents who found the book helpful that we were compelled to write a book specifically for them, called *Smart but Scattered: The Revolutionary "Executive Skills" Approach to Helping Kids Reach Their Potential* (Dawson & Guare, 2009).

We continue to work with students with executive skill weaknesses both in our clinic setting and in the schools in which we consult. And we continue to refine our understanding of how executive skills affect learning and how parents, teachers, and psychologists can intervene effectively. The second edition of this book reflects our evolving understanding of the role executive skills play in academic and social success.

OVERVIEW OF CONTENTS

Chapter 1 defines what we mean by executive skills and lists 11 separate skills included in the construct of executive functioning. This chapter also describes how these skills develop from infancy through adulthood and lists the kinds of developmental tasks for which executive skills are required and the ages at which we expect children to perform such tasks.

Chapter 2 describes the variety of techniques that can be employed to assess executive functioning in children and adolescents, including the use of clinical interviews, behavior rating scales, behavioral observations, and formal test instruments. This chapter features a table that summarizes how each executive skill may appear in testing situations, how it might be displayed on specific tests or subtests, what rating scales may capture the skill, and what it looks like in activities of daily living at home and at school.

Chapter 3 outlines a process for linking assessment to intervention, beginning with the identification of specific skill weaknesses and their behavioral manifestations and leading to the development of multimodal intervention strategies based on the behaviors of concern. It offers sample behavioral objectives developed for each executive skill and a case study illustrating how the assessment process is linked to intervention design. The chapter concludes with an introduction to RTI and how executive skills weaknesses in students can be addressed within a three-tiered model of service delivery.

Chapter 4 broadly overviews intervention strategies that support students with weak executive skills as well as foster the development of more effective skills. Whereas the first edition of this book focused on interventions designed for individual children, we have expanded this chapter to include a discussion of whole-class interventions and of teaching strategies beyond those that address behavioral deficits (such as forgetting to bring home homework assignments at the end of the school day) to include routines to address behavioral excesses, such as poor impulse and emotional control. We also introduce the concept of "scripts" (i.e., self-talk), which has emerged as a promising strategy for improving self-regulation.

Chapter 5 delineates an array of teaching routines that can be used in the classroom either with individual students or whole classes to target common problems associated with weak executive skills. We list the set of steps to follow in teaching the routine, then briefly discuss how the routine can be modified for whole-class use at both the elementary and secondary levels.

Chapter 6 addresses each of the 11 executive functions in turn. We focus both on environmental modifications that can be used to support students with executive skills weaknesses and on strategies for teaching the skill so that students can function independently with respect to the skill in question. Each skill concludes with a vignette that shows how the strategies play out in real-life situations, and a set of "Keys to Success" that reiterate critical aspects of the intervention design that increase the likelihood of improving performance.

Chapter 7 delves into a description of "coaching," an umbrella strategy that we believe has wide application for helping students acquire executive skills. Expanded from the first edition, the chapter includes an overview of research supporting the efficacy of coaching and coaching applications, including peer coaching and group coaching.

Chapter 8 returns to a discussion of executive skills within an RTI model. Whereas Chapter 3 focused on the assessment side of the model, this chapter illuminates the intervention side. Features include a checklist of classroom supports that should be present at Tier 1 (universal level) intervention and a table that lists environmental modifications, instructional supports, and motivational strategies applicable at each of the three tiers. It concludes with a case study of how the RTI process might work with a student with executive skills weaknesses.

Chapter 9 examines executive skills as they may appear in special populations such as children with acquired brain injury, ADHD, and autism spectrum disorders, and we proffer some guidance on how to approach complicated cases, for example, students with multiple learning or behavior problems.

Finally, Chapter 10 proposes ways to handle students with executive skills weaknesses during times of transition. In our work with students, families, and schools, we have found that students are most at risk for regression or failure when they move from grade to grade or from school to school. We offer some suggestions to schools about how to manage these transitions with the hope that all the hard work and success achieved in one school or grade level is not undone in the next.

Contents

Purchasers can download and print copies of the reproducible
materials from *www.guilford.com/dawson3-forms*.

List of Figures and Tables

FIGURES

TABLES

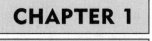

CHAPTER 1

Overview of Executive Skills

Human beings have a built in capacity to meet challenges and accomplish goals through the use of high-level cognitive functions called executive skills. These are the skills that help us to decide what activities or tasks we will pay attention to and which ones we'll choose to do (Hart & Jacobs, 1993). Executive skills allow us to organize our behavior over time and override immediate demands in favor of longer-term goals. Through the use of these skills we can plan and organize activities, sustain attention, and persist to complete a task. Executive skills enable us to manage our emotions and monitor our thoughts in order to work more efficiently and effectively. Simply stated, these skills help us to regulate our behavior.

In a broad sense, executive skills help us to do this in two ways. One way involves the use of certain thinking skills to select and achieve goals or to develop problem solutions. These skills include the following:

- *Planning*—The ability to create a roadmap to reach a goal or to complete a task. It also involves being able to make decisions about what's important to focus on and what's not important.
- *Organization*—The ability to design and maintain systems for keeping track of information or materials.
- *Time management*—The capacity to estimate how much time one has, how to allocate it, and how to stay within time limits and deadlines. It also involves a sense that time is important.
- *Working memory*—The ability to hold information in mind while performing complex tasks. It incorporates the ability to draw on past learning or experience to apply to the situation at hand or to project into the future.
- *Metacognition*—The ability to stand back and take a bird's-eye view of oneself in a situation. It is an ability to observe how you problem solve. It also includes self-monitoring and self-evaluative skills (e.g., asking yourself, "How am I doing?" or "How did I do?").

These skills, then, help us to create a picture of a goal, a path to that goal, and the resources we will need along the way. They also help us to remember the picture even though the goal may be far away and other events come along to occupy our attention and take up space in our memory. But in order to reach the goal we also need to use some other executive skills to guide our behavior as we move along the path. These include the following:

- *Response inhibition*—The capacity to think before you act. This ability to resist the urge to say or do something allows us the time to evaluate a situation and how our behavior might impact it.
- *Emotional control* (also called self-regulation of affect)—The ability to manage emotions in order to achieve goals, complete tasks, or control and direct behavior.
- *Sustained attention*—The capacity to attend to a situation or task in spite of distractibility, fatigue, or boredom.
- *Task initiation*—The ability to begin a task without undue procrastination, in a timely fashion.
- *Flexibility*—The ability to revise plans in the face of obstacles, setbacks, new information, or mistakes. It involves adaptability to changing conditions.
- *Goal directed persistence*—The capacity or drive to follow through to the completion of a goal and not be put off by other demands or competing interests.

When do we need these skills? We don't need them, for the most part, to manage our day-to-day habits and routines. We do need them when we face a new challenge or resolve to pursue a goal.

DEVELOPMENTAL TRENDS

As we noted above, executive skills are built in. But while they are built in, executive skills obviously are not developed at birth, or for some time after that. We see their beginnings in the infant and toddler and even more of them in the 5-year-old. But even in the 15-year-old, we sometimes marvel at the lack of planning, time management, or especially inhibition. So these skills, which are at the heart of self-regulation or self-control, begin to develop in early infancy and continue to develop well into adolescence and early adulthood. If we can understand how these skills improve through childhood, we can begin to understand how much control children exercise over themselves at different ages. This information in turn can help us as adults to know how much support and structure to provide as children develop.

EXECUTIVE SKILLS AND BRAIN DEVELOPMENT

Before we consider the developmental sequence, however, we need to look briefly at the way executive skills relate to the brain and brain development. At birth, the child's brain weighs about 400 grams. By late adolescence this has increased to about 1,400 grams (Kolb

& Wishaw, 1990), or from 10–12 ounces to a little over 3 pounds. A number of changes in the brain account for this significant growth. Broadly speaking, growth of the brain over the course of development occurs through the generation of nerve cells (neurons) and their supporting cells (neuroglia). These cells are the building blocks of the nervous system. In order for nerve cells to "talk" with each other, they develop branches, called axons and dendrites, which allow them to send and receive information from other cells.

When we talk about the material that makes up the brain—neurons, dendrites, axons, and so forth—we can think about this in terms of shadings of the brain; that is, gray and white matter. The white matter of the brain acquires its shading through a process called myelination and represents bundles of axons that connect different regions of the brain and allows them to communicate. Myelin is a fatty sheath that forms around the axon and provides insulation that helps to increase speed of transmission of nerve signals. Thus, the "conversations" (as nerve signals) carried by axons between neurons are made more efficient by this process of insulation. Myelination begins in the earliest stages of development and in the frontal lobes continues well into young adulthood. This process is one of the key features of frontal lobe development, and the time course of this process parallels the time course and development of executive skills.

Gray matter, in contrast to the white matter of myelin, is made up of nerve cells or neurons and the connections between them are called synapses. Unlike myelin, the development of gray matter is a bit more complex, involving a series of increases followed by reductions. For example, it is estimated that the fetal brain, at 5 months' gestation, has about 100 billion neurons. This is comparable to the number of neurons in the average adult brain. And in early childhood, the number of synapses (about a quadrillion) greatly exceeds the number in the adult brain. If the development of gray matter continued at this pace, the adult brain would be enormous. Instead, a different phenomenon occurs. There is an initial increase in gray matter (neurons and particularly synapses) in early childhood. This increase peaks before age 5 and then there is a gradual reduction or "pruning" of these connections. The initial increase occurs during a period of rapid learning and experience in early childhood. Recent brain research suggests that as this learning and skill development becomes more efficient, additional increases in gray matter could actually undermine new learning. The pruning process allows the child to consolidate skills, and the gray matter connections that are not needed or used drop away. This period of consolidation continues until a second period of significant growth in gray matter begins around age 11 or 12, the onset of another period that we recognize for rapid learning and development. This increase is again followed by a period of reduction through pruning over the course of adolescence.

Research indicates that this growth spurt in the brain prior to adolescence occurs primarily in the frontal lobes. Thus, it is as if the brain is preparing itself both for the development of executive skills as well as for the significant demands that will be made on executive skills during adolescence. Researchers at the National Institute of Mental Health also suggest that a "use it or lose it" process may be occurring in the frontal lobes during this time. Neural connections that are used are retained, while those that are not exercised are lost. If this is the case, then not only is the practice of these skills important for learning self-management, but also for the development of brain structures that will support these skills into later adolescence and adulthood. During this period, teachers and parents can play a critical role in guiding the learning and development of executive skills.

Thus, there is a parallel between development of the brain and development of the child's ability to act, think, and feel. This parallel is especially important in understanding how executive skills develop and what areas of the brain are most critical for these skills. Researchers now generally agree that frontal brain systems (the frontal/prefrontal cortex along with connections to adjacent areas) make up the neurological base for executive skills. Figure 1.1 depicts the human brain with the approximate location of major functions, including executive skills in the prefrontal cortex.

We do not mean to oversimplify or suggest that the prefrontal cortex is the only area of the brain related to executive skills. Recent neuroimaging evidence suggests that other areas of the brain also are involved (Pliszka, 2002). Nonetheless, the prefrontal cortex and nearby associated systems play a pre-eminent role in the relationship between brain structure and executive function.

Prefrontal brain systems are among the last to fully develop, in late adolescence, and they are the final, common pathway for managing information and behavior from other brain regions. Hart and Jacobs (1993) have summarized the critical functions of the frontal lobes in the management of information and behavior:

1. The frontal lobes decide what is worth attending to and what is worth doing.
2. The frontal lobes provide continuity and coherence to behavior across time.

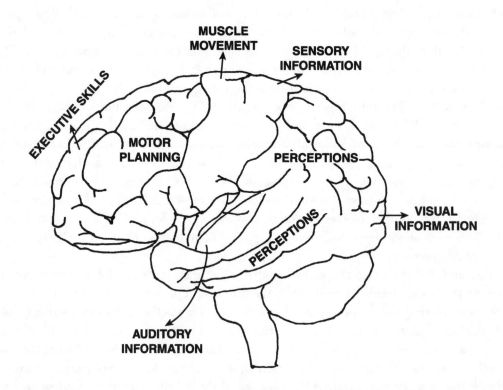

FIGURE 1.1. The human brain, with the approximate location of major functions.

3. The frontal lobes modulate affective and interpersonal behaviors so that drives are satisfied within the constraints of the internal and external environments.
4. The frontal lobes monitor, evaluate, and adjust. (pp. 2, 3)

Thus, the executive skills we have defined above are intimately tied to the frontal lobes and more broadly to frontal brain systems. This relationship can help us understand how executive skills develop over the course of childhood. It can also help us understand how executive skills can be affected by factors such as attention deficit disorder or brain injury.

SEQUENCE OF DEVELOPMENT

At birth we do not have executive skills that are developed or available for use. Instead, they lie dormant in the brain as future skills, in much the same way language does. Assuming there is no insult to the brain and that experience is reasonably normal, these skills will unfold over time. But as they unfold, they are influenced by the genes that we inherit from our parents as well as by the biological and social environment in which we live. If our parents did not have good organization or attention skills, chances are increased that we will have executive skill problems. If we are raised in a biologically or socially toxic environment, for example, where lead exposure or psychological trauma takes place, there is an increased likelihood that executive skills will suffer. However, assuming that no genetic or environmental disasters take place, executive skills will begin to develop and show themselves soon after birth in a slow progression to full adult development.

Of the theories of executive function, we favor the model proposed by Barkley (1997) since he attempts to provide a sequence for the development of these skills beginning in infancy (Figure 1.2). Barkley's model contains five essential elements: behavioral inhibition; working memory (nonverbal); internalization of speech (verbal working memory); self-regulation of affect/motivation/arousal; and reconstitution (Barkley, 1997, p. 191). The cornerstone of this model is behavioral inhibition, which begins to emerge in the 5- to 12-month age range. This first executive function has three properties that allow us to delay or stop a behavior:

1. *The ability to delay or prevent the response leading to an immediate consequence so that some later occurring consequence may impact behavior* ("I won't make this sarcastic comment now that would annoy my teacher. I'll listen quietly so she'll respond positively to me later").
2. *The ability to stop ongoing behaviors when they prove unsuccessful* ("The comments I'm making are not getting a positive response from my teacher").
3. *The ability to manage distractions or interruptions that could interfere with the work of other executive skills* ("I need to move away from my friend because his comments are distracting me from keeping in mind what my teacher is saying").

Thus, *behavioral inhibition* helps us to think before we act and to decide when and if we will respond. It precedes the other executive functions and shields them from interference.

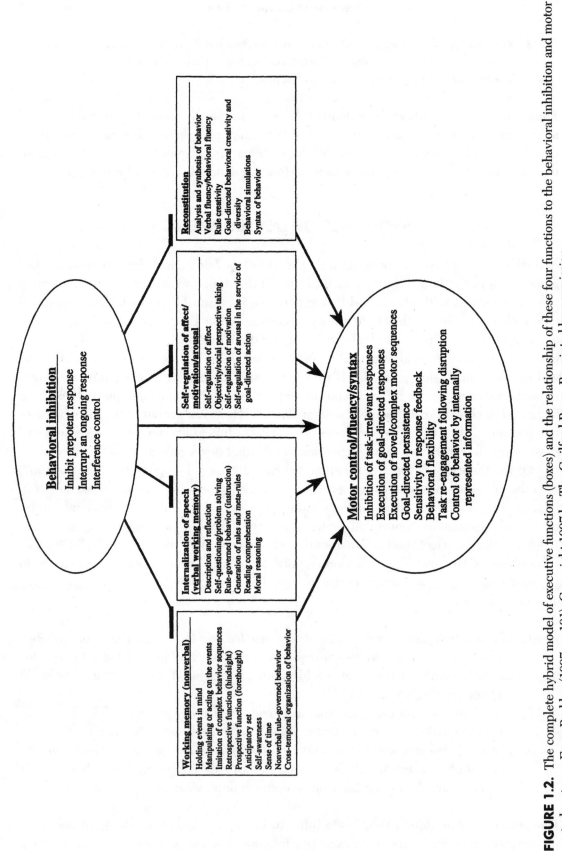
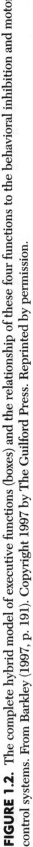

FIGURE 1.2. The complete hybrid model of executive functions (boxes) and the relationship of these four functions to the behavioral inhibition and motor control systems. From Barkley (1997, p. 191). Copyright 1997 by The Guilford Press. Reprinted by permission.

If we didn't have inhibition, it is easy to see that our ability to use planning, goal-directed persistence, and so on would be very difficult. For the infant, inhibition is the first and most basic step in self-control because it gives the infant the power to respond or not respond to a person or event. Throughout life we use this ability to stop or delay a response as a way both to manage our own behavior and to influence the behavior of others.

While behavioral inhibition gives the infant some control over what to respond to (e.g., "I can respond or not respond to this person in front of me making the funny face"), the infant remains stuck in the present. Without some type of memory, some ability to represent real people and events in the mind, the infant can only respond to what he or she can see/hear/touch and so on, right now, in this place right here. This sets the stage for the next executive skill in the Barkley model: *nonverbal working memory*. Development of this skill begins in the 5- to 12-month age range and involves the ability to hold information "on line" in the mind. This gives the infant the rudimentary capacity to move beyond "right now" and "right here." Nonverbal working memory becomes the foundation for the child's ability to make decisions and control behavior even though a person or an activity is not present here or now. As information and experience increase, the child develops the ability to look backward and forward ("hindsight" and "forethought"; Barkley, 1997, pp. 165–166), to mentally manipulate events, and to imitate more complex behaviors. With the expansion of his or her mental life, the child becomes less tied to the events and consequences of the immediate situation, of here-and-now "real life." Because of this, behavior can be brought under control of mental representations ("Last Saturday, after I finished cleaning my room, mom took me and a friend out for pizza. I'll ask her if we can do that again after I clean my room"). Obviously the infant does not have this capacity but, in the ability to hold a picture of the mother in his or her mind, we can see the beginnings of this control.

Internalization of speech is the next of the executive skills to develop according to Barkley (1997, p. 174). Acquisition of language provides the child with a powerful tool for control of the environment. People, objects, and actions and the images of these that the child has formed in nonverbal working memory can now be represented with words. More important, these words provide the child with a means for exercising some control over the world. It is no longer necessary for the child to walk to his or her mother or point to what he or she wants. Instead the child can use words to accomplish what previously took physical actions. Language also becomes an increasingly powerful means for adults (and other children) to regulate the child's behavior. What begins as management of behavior by the language of other people gradually shifts in part to self-management. Initially, the child accomplishes this by adopting the adult words and publicly saying them to him- or herself. According to Barkley, this self-speech is evident in the 3- to 5-year-old and becomes increasingly more private or covert until it is largely internalized by 9–12 years. This skill involves much more than basic self-control. Over time, internalization of speech facilitates the development of rules, problem-solving strategies, self-monitoring, self-instruction, and metacognition.

The fourth skill in Barkley's model is self-regulation of affect/motivation/arousal (Barkley, 1997, p. 211). The earliest manifestation of this skill comes in the 5-month range and becomes more evident when locomotion develops. It involves a number of subskills including regulation of emotional and motivational states, regulation of arousal, and the capacity for social perspective taking. We can begin to see how the development of this skill can give emotional and motivational value to the mental representations that the child is forming in working memory. Initially, for example, the child sees the mother's face and associates this stimulus with a feeling of pleasure or comfort. With the representation of mother's face in working memory, the child can experience the pleasure in the absence of the "real" stimulus and be motivated/aroused to seek the mother. Thus, the pleasurable representation triggers a drive that leads to a motor response. Behavioral inhibition may come into play when the child crosses paths with a potentially distracting stimulus (e.g., a favored toy), but is able to ignore this and continue in pursuit of the original goal. As the child's representational experiences grow and acquire emotional value, and as hindsight and forethought expand across time, choices multiply and the child is freed from control by the immediate environment. Longer-term goals (from the infant's search for the mother to the teenager's search for a college) become increasingly more powerful factors in setting a behavioral direction. Language is the next factor to significantly enhance this capacity.

The final element to develop in the Barkley model is reconstitution, defined as the "analysis and synthesis of behavior" (1997, p. 185). This executive skill enables the individual to divide more complex behavioral sequences into component units (analysis) and recombine them in novel ways (synthesis) to solve new problems or reach new goals. Hence, reconstitution represents cognitive and behavioral flexibility, fluency, and creativity. Barkley sees this skill as representing the capacity for covert rehearsal or simulation before making a decision on how best to proceed. Thus, it is an opportunity for the child to find a good fit between a problem or goal and a behavioral strategy. This obviously is a more sophisticated and later-developing skill that, based on research about children's planning ability, emerges in its early stages at about 6 years.

These skills, then, are critical if children are to develop complex independent living and problem-solving abilities. Although executive skills begin to emerge in early infancy, they reach a reasonable level of development only by mid-to-late adolescence. It is at this point that relevant adults (e.g., parents, teachers, employers) begin to feel more confidence in the self-regulatory ability of the teenager. This increased confidence is reflected in the choices and opportunities that we make available such as a driver's license, less restricted work hours, course selection, and credit cards. Prior to this development, adults help compensate for incomplete development by "lending" their frontal lobes or executive skills to the child.

This happens in one of two ways. The first is direct, coming in the form of directives, limits, and rules. For example, in the toddler who has little impulse control, moving toward potential danger typically leads to a sharp "No!" Or for the young child who is unable to make and follow a plan, we, the adults, construct the plan and then prompt or cue each step, not completing the task for the child but ensuring that with help they are successful. In effect, we are a surrogate frontal lobe that operates for the child as a set of supplementary executive skills. However, we are not there indefinitely to provide these skills. Rather, we are there to prompt and to teach them, and then to step back as the child's own executive skills unfold.

The second method involves structuring the environment in a way that compensates for underdeveloped skills. For example, with a toddler we use gates to prohibit entry or escape. We order the environment and label it with pictures or words to help organization.

For the adolescent we gate off, as best we can, access to alcohol, drugs, and weapons. And we attempt to hold them in a controlled environment—school—where their options only gradually expand. This model is not universal, but it certainly prevails in western cultures (and gradually emerges in developing countries).

DEVELOPMENTAL TASKS REQUIRING EXECUTIVE SKILLS

Let's move from theory to a concrete description of the kinds of tasks children and teenagers perform that require executive skills. Table 1.1 lists specific tasks or behaviors adults commonly expect children to be able to perform in different age ranges. In reviewing this table, the reader should keep in mind that there are developmental variations between children such that at any given age some children can perform tasks at an independent level while other children will require cuing, supervision, or even assistance to perform the same tasks. This table should be considered as approximate rather than explicit guidelines for behavioral expectations at any age level.

Determining the level of a child's executive skills in relation to these developmental tasks can help us to understand the "goodness of fit" between the child and his or her world. This assessment in turn can help us to judge the adjustments that may be needed in the degree of "frontal lobe" support provided by adults, whether modifications in adult expectations are called for, and whether environmental supports should be added or withdrawn. Such an assessment also sets the stage for determining the next set of skills to be taught as well as how these executive skills can be shaped to promote both success and independence.

TABLE 1.1. Developmental Tasks Requiring Executive Skills

Age range	Developmental task
Preschool	Run simple errands (e.g., "Get your shoes from the bedroom").
	Tidy bedroom or playroom with assistance.
	Perform simple chores and self-help tasks with reminders (e.g., clear dishes from table, brush teeth, get dressed).
	Inhibit behaviors: don't touch a hot stove, run into the street, grab a toy from another child, hit, bite, push, etc.
Kindergarten–grade 2	Run errands (two- to three-step directions).
	Tidy bedroom or playroom.
	Perform simple chores, self-help tasks; may need reminders (e.g., make bed).
	Bring papers to and from school.
	Complete homework assignments (20 minutes maximum).
	Decide how to spend money (allowance).
	Inhibit behaviors: follow safety rules, don't swear, raise hand before speaking in class, keep hands to self.
Grades 3–5	Run errands (may involve time delay or greater distance, such as going to a nearby store or remembering to do something after school).
	Tidy bedroom or playroom (may include vacuuming, dusting, etc.).
	Perform chores that take 15–30 minutes (e.g., clean up after dinner, rake leaves).
	Bring books, papers, assignments to and from school.
	Keep track of belongings when away from home.
	Complete homework assignments (1 hour maximum).
	Plan simple school project such as book report (select book, read book, write report).
	Keep track of changing daily schedule (i.e., different activities after school).
	Save money for desired objects, plan how to earn money.
	Inhibit/self-regulate: behave when teacher is out of the classroom; refrain from rude comments, temper tantrums, bad manners.
Grades 6–8	Help out with chores around the home, including both daily responsibilities and occasional tasks (e.g., emptying dishwasher, raking leaves, shoveling snow); tasks may take 60–90 minutes to complete.
	Babysit younger siblings or for pay.
	Use system for organizing schoolwork; including assignment book, notebooks, etc.
	Follow complex school schedule involving changing teachers and changing schedules.
	Plan and carry out long-term projects, including tasks to be accomplished and reasonable timeline to follow; may require planning multiple large projects simultaneously.
	Plan time, including after-school activities, homework, family responsibilities; estimate how long it takes to complete individual tasks and adjust schedule to fit.
	Inhibit rule breaking in the absence of visible authority.

(cont.)

TABLE 1.1. *(cont.)*

Age range	Developmental task
High school	Manage schoolwork effectively on a day-to-day basis, including completing and handing in assignments on time, studying for tests, creating and following timelines for long-term projects, and making adjustments in effort and quality of work in response to feedback from teachers and others (e.g., grades on tests, papers).
	Establish and refine a long-term goal and make plans for meeting that goal. If the goal beyond high school is college, the youngster selects appropriate courses and maintains GPA to ensure acceptance into college. The youngster also participates in extracurricular activities, signs up for and takes SATs or ACTs at the appropriate time and carries out the college application process. If the youngster does not plan to go to college, he or she pursues vocational courses and, if applicable, employment outside of school to ensure the training and experience necessary to obtain employment after graduation.
	Make good use of leisure time, including obtaining employment or pursuing recreational activities during the summer.
	Inhibit reckless and dangerous behaviors (e.g., use of illegal substances, sexual acting out, shoplifting, vandalism).

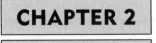

CHAPTER 2

Assessing Executive Skills

For those who are accustomed to using standardized measures to assess processing disorders or learning disabilities, the assessment of executive functions presents a somewhat different challenge. It is possible to assess language-based learning disorders, nonverbal learning disabilities, and dyslexia using instruments such as tests of intelligence, achievement, language, memory, and phonological processing—tests that are normed on a typical population of students—with a diagnosis deriving from a distinct cognitive profile.

Although efforts have been made to develop formal measures of executive functioning in children, many have argued that the efforts have fallen short for a number of reasons. Anderson (1998) pointed out that those tests that are most available for assessing executive skills in children were developed originally for use with an adult population and because they were not designed with children in mind they may lack both appeal as well as sufficient normative information. Since they were designed for use with a clinical population (e.g., head injured), they fail to take into account the normal developmental progression of executive skills in childhood. Furthermore, the tasks developed often require the child to use other skills, such as language, memory, and motor functioning, that confound the test results—does the child have difficulty copying a complex visual design because of poor planning or organization (two executive skills) or because of poor motor control, for instance. Others (e.g., Isquith, Crawford, Espy, & Gioia, 2005) have raised questions about the ecological validity of clinic measures of executive skills. As Isquith et al. point out, "An ecologically valid assessment tool is one that has characteristics similar to a naturally occurring behavior and has value in predicting everyday function" (p. 210). When performance-based tests are designed to ensure internal validity, the result is tests that "assess more narrow, situationally constrained processes in contrast to real-world adaptive executive functions" (p. 210).

Attempting to assess executive skills in the context of a formal evaluation is difficult because so many of the factors that demand the use of executive skills on the part of the student are removed from the equation. Just some examples of why this is the case:

- Two critical executive skills are initiation and sustained attention. In standardized testing situations, the examiner cues the student to start and presents task that are necessarily brief in nature, thereby reducing the demand for sustained attention.
- Standardized testing situations require the presence of an adult performing a monitoring function. With the evaluator performing this role, the student does not have to monitor his or her own performance to the same extent, a critical executive skill.
- In the context of a highly structured, if not ritualized, set of tasks, the need for planning and organization on the part of the student is reduced, if not in many cases eliminated.
- Executive skills are most in demand in the face of complex, open-ended tasks requiring problem solving and creative or unique solutions. Standardized tests are designed to be easily scored with a catalog of right and wrong answers that are straightforward and invariant, again minimizing demands on executive skills.
- The most complex cognitive task within any psychologist's repertoire is less complex than real-world demands on executive skills, and there is no way of determining with any certainty how well these tests map on to the real world. Thus, in the parlance of neuropsychologists, *absence of evidence is not evidence of absence.* In other words, a child's strong performance on a clinic measure of executive function (such as the Porteus Mazes) does not necessarily mean that that same child applies good planning ability in the context of daily performance at home or at school.

IS THERE A PLACE FOR THE USE OF FORMAL ASSESSMENT MEASURES?

Proponents of response to intervention (RTI) have argued forcefully that there is no place for cognitive testing in determining whether a student has a learning disability (e.g., Gresham, Restori, & Cook, 2008), and therefore much of the IQ testing that school psychologists do is unnecessary and takes time that could be better spent on other activities that research shows benefit students. We agree that academic skill deficits are better assessed directly, and that curriculum-based measurement (CBM) is the best methodology both for identifying delays in academic skill acquisition and in measuring progress and efficacy of interventions. CBM is not designed to measure executive skills, however, and yet no experienced teacher or parent would deny the impact of executive skills on academic skill acquisition and school performance. For this reason, behavior rating scale results and careful interviews conducted with parents and teachers are most likely to yield useful and reliable information about the impact of executive skill weaknesses on everyday performance, both at home and at school.

Despite the limitations of formal assessment, we have found it useful in our practice to allocate a portion of the assessment process to direct work with children, and more often than not this involves the use of formal assessment measures. In addition to providing, for example, information about a child's cognitive functioning, these kinds of tests present the opportunity to engage in a structured observation of the child performing tasks that appear to have some face validity with respect to executive skills. Cognitive and neuropsychological tests, such as the NEPSY-II, present students with a structured set of tasks, graded for difficulty level so that the challenge increases as each test or subtest progresses. Some of these tasks are appealing, some are less so. Observing how children respond to the increasing challenge, which demands that they shift quickly from one task to another and that they employ some kind of problem-solving strategy, gives us some insight into their ability to deploy efficiently a number of executive skills, particularly response inhibition, emotional control, flexibility, and metacognition. While there are limitations to our ability to observe these behaviors in one-on-one testing situations, the glimpses we get are invaluable in helping us "fill out the picture."

We should note that we collect rating scales and conduct parent and/or teacher interviews prior to working with children. Thus, we approach the assessment not only with a great deal of background information but also having formulated some hypotheses about executive functioning and particular executive skill weaknesses affecting school performance. This means we can carefully select instruments designed to test those hypotheses, enabling us to make efficient use of the time we have available for working with children directly.

Furthermore, this direct interaction with children allows us to get to know a child in a richer and more nuanced way than would be possible if we were only looking at behavior counts or even basing our understanding of the child on classroom observations. In our clinical experience both parents and teachers tend to be skeptical when we attempt to render judgments about a child without taking the time to get to know the child in question.

Certainly for children with mild executive skill weaknesses, a comprehensive assessment, such as that described above and in the table at the end of this chapter, is likely unnecessary, and a graduated assessment method, such as that incorporated in RTI as it is commonly used, is recommended. For more complex problems or situations where parents and teachers are confused or do not agree on the nature of the problem, pulling together information from a variety of sources and methods makes sense to us.

COMPONENTS OF THE ASSESSMENT PROCESS

Best practice in the assessment of executive function must extend beyond the use of formal standardized measures. While we believe such measures may have a place in the evaluation process, several additional sources of information are also critical when a comprehensive assessment is desired (1) a detailed case history with interview questions designed to elicit the presence or absence of executive skills in everyday activities; (2) standardized behavior rating scales; (3) classroom observations; and (4) work samples. These elements are discussed below.

Informal Assessment Measures

Case History/Interview

A critical piece of the process when assessing a youngster's executive functioning is to gather information from those who know the child best, usually parents and teachers. When we interview parents, we ask questions about how children manage homework and other chores and responsibilities at home. For instance, can they plan tasks on their own, do they need reminders to get started on homework, do they need encouragement to keep working until the job is done, and do they need constant supervision to ensure task completion? How do they handle morning or bedtime routines: can they follow them independently or do they need cues and reminders? We ask how organized they are: Do they keep their bedrooms or study areas neat, do they know where to find belongings, do they keep notebooks and back-packs organized? And we ask questions about their ability to control their behavior—with friends, with siblings, with parents, when frustrated, when stressed, when disappointed. All of these questions tell us something about youngsters' ability to plan and organize, initiate tasks, and sustain attention, as well as their ability to regulate their behavior when confronted with obstacles.

Teachers can provide us similar information. When we interview teachers, we ask them how well the student in question is able to work independently, how well he or she organizes and keeps track of materials and possessions in school, and how well he or she plans and executes activities. And, again, we ask about his or her ability to manage behavior when stressed and his or her ability to control impulses.

We ask older students (and some more insightful younger ones) similar questions. We inquire about common homework problems, their ability to plan for long-term projects, how they study for tests, and what organizational strategies they use to keep track of things. We also ask about leisure time activities. Do they use their time well or do they tend to spend too much time engaged in any activity—hanging out with friends, instant messaging, playing computer and video games? We may also ask them how they manage negative emotions. Do siblings, parents, or other kids get on their nerves, what do they do when an assignment frustrates them, and so on?

The objective is to complete a mini-functional assessment to determine (1) specific behaviors that demonstrate strong/weak executive skills; (2) circumstances (people, places, times) under which the problems are most/least likely to occur; (3) previous successful/unsuccessful interventions; and (4) capacity/receptivity of the people and/or environment to change. Obviously not all questions may be answered during the interview but in the same sense that the assessment process leads to generation and clarification of hypotheses about skills, it also leads to generation and clarification of possible interventions. For example, knowing that a parent is organizationally challenged or that a teacher already feels overwhelmed by demands on his or her time can lead to different decisions about intervention.

The Appendix contains structured interview forms that can be used with parents, teachers, and students to assess executive skills. (See Forms 2.1, 2.2, and 2.3 on pp. 169, 173, 177.) The questions on all three questionnaires are organized around common problem areas that students have rather than around specific executive skills deficits. However, to facilitate identifying specific executive skills deficits each question is coded with the executive skill it is believed to tap. These three sources provide us with rich clinical data about how parents, teachers, and youngsters themselves view executive functioning. From this data alone, we can begin to formulate some environmental modifications and behavioral interventions, but we find it helpful to add normative data to this mix as well.

Classroom Observations

Classroom observation can play a key role in assessment and intervention since it provides the opportunity to see executive skills in their most important context—the daily demands of school. It is within the setting of the classroom environment or classroom demands (e.g., homework) that executive skills problems often are first noted and the success of any intervention will be judged by an observed change in behavior. Hence, a classroom observation sets the stage for a clear definition of the executive skill as a specific behavior, points to the direction for intervention, and provides the gold standard for evaluating effectiveness (i.e., did the behavior change?). In conducting the observation, the setting events, antecedents, and responses to the behavior may all be visible to the observer, along with the impact of potential interventions (Figure 2.1).

A second alternative is to have the teacher, aide, or another specialist (e.g., school psychologist, counselor, occupational therapist) collect some of the data. For this to be feasible, data collection methods need to fit easily with the schedule of the classroom and the

---

- Complete interviews and rating scales prior to scheduling the classroom observation. This gives the evaluator a good idea about the problem areas and in what classroom situations they are likely to be observed.
- Identify with the classroom teacher what his or her primary concerns are and identify the times or classroom activities in which the behaviors of concern are most likely to be observed. Let the teacher know whether he or she should intervene as is typically done (e.g., redirecting the child to get back to work) or if the teacher should not intervene so that the observer can get an idea of how the child behaves when left "on his or her own."
- Sit behind the target child or off to the side, in a location where the child cannot make easy eye contact with the observer.
- Collect both objective data (e.g., percent of time on task) as well as a running record of the child's behavior throughout the observation.
- In addition to observing the child, observe the physical environment to determine if there are factors about the classroom space that might be contributing to the problem or could be changed to reduce the problem. Watch the teacher to see how he or she cues the child or manages the classroom routines. This information could prove valuable when planning interventions.
- Arrange, if time permits, to come back and observe on another day. Several short observations spread over several days may be more useful than one long observation on a single day.
- Be sure to check back with the teacher after the observation to determine whether the behavior observed was typical or atypical of the child.
- Observe the child in settings other than the classroom. This is particularly important if the child's problems relate to poor impulse control or regulation of affect, since these behaviors are likely to be more evident in less structured situations such as in the hallways, in the cafeteria, or out at recess.

FIGURE 2.1. Tips for doing classroom observations.

person observing, particularly if it is the teacher. Fortunately, a number of executive skills involve production (homework, classwork, projects) so that work samples (see below for more details) or the absence of them are a readily available "permanent product measure" that can be used to assess behavior. For other executive skill weaknesses, the type of behavior will determine the observation method. For example, the length of time needed to begin a task, the percent of time on task, and the number of times speaking out will serve as reliable measures of task initiation, sustained attention, and response inhibition, respectively.

As noted above, observed behavior or its product in natural, everyday settings ultimately will constitute the best measure of an executive skill. A change in the behavior will constitute the best measure of an effective intervention. Prior to intervention, the person seeking the change (parent, teacher, student) must come to an agreement with the person planning the intervention about what outcome behavior will need to be observed to define success.

Work Samples

Work samples such as tests, writing assignments, and agenda pages can help assess skills such as error monitoring, planning, and organization, as well as yield ideas for interventions such as cue questions and templates. Work samples might also include looking at the child's backpack or desk to get a better sense of the child's ability to organize his or her personal space.

Behavior Checklists

Behavior checklists serve two functions in our assessment of executive skills. First of all, the use of broad-band instruments, such as the Achenbach scales or the Behavior Assessment System for Children, Second Edition (BASC-2), provide a picture of the child's social–emotional adjustment in general. Executive skill weaknesses can often be associated with a variety of disorders, such as anxiety, depression, and disruptive behavior disorders, and this gives us a larger context within which to understand executive functioning. It also facilitates differential diagnosis, enabling a deeper understanding of the factors that might be affecting the child's overall adjustment. Second, behavior rating scales give us a picture of the child's executive functioning in everyday activities. Given the limitations to formal assessment of executive skills, this is a critical piece in our assessment process. A sample of available rating scales, both broad- or narrow-band, are discussed below.

Behavior Rating Inventory of Executive Functions

Available from Psychological Assessment Resources (PAR), the Behavior Rating Inventory of Executive Functions (BRIEF) was normed on children ages 6–18 and includes both parent and teacher versions (Gioia, Isquith, Guy, and Kenworthy, 2000). It is an 86-item inventory in which the parent or teacher is asked to determine on a 3-point scale how often the child performs the problem behavior (never, sometimes, always). The scale yields a global measure of executive functioning as well as two indexes, Behavioral Regulation and Metacognition, and eight scales assessing individual executive skills. The Behavioral Regulation Index includes three subscales, Inhibit, Shift, and Emotional Control, while the Metacognition Index includes five scales: Initiate, Working Memory, Plan/Organize, Organization of Materials, and Monitor.

There are two additional versions of the BRIEF for children, a preschool version (BRIEF-P), normed on children ages 2–5 (both parent and teacher norms) and a self-report version (BRIEF-SR), normed on children ages 11–18. We have found the BRIEF-P very helpful, particularly in identifying children with weaknesses in emotional control and flexibility. Our experience with the self-report form is that children have a tendency to under-report problems compared to parent and teacher reports. We are most likely to use this checklist after working with or interviewing the youngster and gauging his or her ability to respond honestly to the items.

Brown Attention-Deficit Disorder Scales for Children and Adolescents

Available from Pearson Education (Brown, 1996, 2001), these rating scales are designed for multiple uses, including screening, as part of a comprehensive diagnosis of attention-deficit/hyperactivity disorder (ADHD), and for monitoring treatment responses. Parent and teacher forms are available for ages 3–7 and 8–12, and self-report versions are available for ages 8–12 and 12–18. The adolescent version yields five cluster scores (Activation, Attention, Effort, Affect, and Memory), while the younger versions add a sixth cluster score assessing "self-regulating action."

Child Behavior Checklist—Teacher Report Form

Both the Child Behavior Checklist (CBCL) and the Teacher Report Form (TRF) were developed by Thomas M. Achenbach (1991a, 1991b) and his colleagues and are designed as broad measures of social–emotional functioning. Checklist items are scored according to broad clusters (Total Problems, Externalizing Problems, and Internalizing Problems) as well as individual scales. Both parent and teacher versions are available, with a preschool version (1.5–5 years) and school-age version (6–18 years), as well as a self-report version (12–18 years). Specific items tap executive skills, particularly those included on the Attention Problems scale. In addition, however, these measures are useful for the open-ended questions included on the form. For instance, the Teacher Report Form asks the teacher to indicate both the "best things about this pupil," and "what concerns you most about this pupil?" Answers to these questions can provide insight into the teacher's perceptions of a child's executive skills depending on the nature of the responses.

Behavior Assessment System for Children, Second Edition

The BASC-2 is another set of rating scales designed to assess behaviors and emotional functioning at the preschool, child, and adolescent level, and include parent, teacher, and self-report versions. Scoring the checklist produces composite scales (e.g., Adaptive Skills,

Behavioral Symptoms Index, Externalizing Problems, Internalizing Problems) as well as individual clinical and adaptive scales. The computer scoring package also yields additional Content Scales, including ones for Executive Functioning and Emotional Self-Control.

Executive Skills Questionnaire for Parents/Teachers and Students

We have developed our own brief rating scale—the Executive Skills Questionnaire (ESQ)—that parents, teachers, and older students can complete to provide additional information regarding executive skill strengths and weaknesses. These can be found in the Appendix. (See Forms 2.4 and 2.5 on pp. 183, 185.) These are not a norm-referenced instrument and should not replace the use of norm-referenced rating scales. We include them for several reasons. First of all, they are aligned with the specific executive skills presented in this manual, thus making it easier to link assessment to the interventions we describe in later chapters. Second, whereas most behavior rating scales, including the BRIEF, focus on areas of weakness, the ESQ enables the evaluator to identify both areas of strength and areas of weakness. Third, we believe that the student version of this instrument can be used not only to help students better understand the nature of their own executive skill strengths and weaknesses, but it also can be used by teachers when making grouping decisions for group learning activities (discussed more in Chapter 4). The parent/teacher version we have included in the appendix is a generic one, intended for children of school age and appropriate for both parents and teachers to complete. Our book *Smart but Scattered* (Dawson & Guare, 2009) includes several versions for children at different ages (preschool, lower elementary, upper elementary, middle school). The student version is intended for use with middle and high school students.

Assessment Rubrics

Another informal way to assess executive skills, both as a means of assessing baseline performance as well as monitoring progress over time, is through the use of rubrics. Figure 2.2 depicts a rubric developed by teachers at Cape Elizabeth High School in Cape Elizabeth, Maine. The rubric is designed for both self-assessment by the student as well as by teachers. Thus, it offers the opportunity to give students a "reality check" so they can see whether their own assessment of executive skill capacity matches up against the perception of their teachers.

Formal Assessment Measures

Formal assessment serves a number of functions. It provides the context for examining other variables such as cognitive abilities, emotional status, and academic skills that may well impact and be impacted by executive skills. In complex cases (see Chapter 9) formal assessment can play a key role in intervention planning and prioritization, in some cases, relegating executive skill problems to the "back burner" until more significant factors are addressed. Formal assessment also can provide a mini laboratory, allowing the evaluator

Student Name: _____ Date: _____ Class: _____

Criteria	Expert (4)	Advanced (3)	Developing (2)	Novice (1)	Student	Teacher
Materials	Brings all necessary materials to class on a daily basis plus additional learning aids (highlighters, etc.).	Often brings all necessary materials to class.	Materials are sometimes missing. Occasionally asks to go to locker to retrieve materials (no more than three times per term).	Materials are frequently missing. Must ask to borrow writing utensils, paper, or copies of handouts or go to locker to retrieve materials (more than three times per term).		
Organization	Materials are complete, neatly organized, well maintained, and modified to assist in learning.	Materials are complete, neatly organized, and well maintained.	Materials are complete but not neatly organized or well maintained.	Materials are incomplete or disorganized.		
Promptness	Independently arrives to class or appointments on time or early every day.	Frequently arrives to class or appointments on time. Is not tardy to class more than three times per term and has pass explaining legitimate reason.	Arrives to class or appointments on time. Is not tardy to class more than five times per term and has pass explaining reason although may not seem legitimate.	Is often tardy to class or appointments more than five times per term. Rarely has a legitimate reason.		
Assignment completion	Assignments are ready to be handed in before the due date. Often makes use of teacher or supports to edit work when needed.	Assignments are handed in on time, when requested during class. Occasionally makes use of teacher or supports to edit work when needed.	Assignments are ready to be handed in but forgotten in locker, at home, or other excuse. Rarely makes use of teacher or supports to edit work when needed.	Assignments are passed in after due date. Does not make use of teacher or supports to edit work.		
Note taking	Independently identifies important concepts and includes them into notes, which are accurate and complete. Frequently reorganizes and/or reviews notes in order to assist with learning.	Identifies some important concepts and includes them into notes, which are somewhat accurate and complete. Occasionally reorganizes and/or reviews notes.	Rarely identifies important concepts and produces notes that are incomplete or not thorough enough to aid in learning. Rarely reorganizes and/or reviews notes.	Seems unable to identify important concepts. Notes are incomplete or not taken. Does not reorganize or review notes.		
Homework completion	Independently completes all homework and often does extra work to further learning rather than for a grade.	Completes homework assignments and occasionally does extra work to further learning.	Homework is incomplete (at least three times per term) and rarely does extra work.	Homework is rarely completed or passed in (more than three times per term) and does not engage in extra work.		

20

Flexibility	Able to multitask or transition between many activities without anxiety. Is always able to adjust to changes in plan, schedule, or due dates without issue.	Able to shift from one activity to another without anxiety. Is mostly able to adjust to changes in plan, schedule, or due dates without issue.	Unable to transition to different activities without experiencing anxiety. May have difficulty adjusting to changes in plan, schedule, or due dates.	Experiences anxiety during any transition or sudden change. Is unable to adjust to changes in plan, schedule, or due dates without significant issue.
Work habits	Is "on task" and works until the end of class, will remain after class to finish work, or takes work home. Makes frequent thoughtful contributions to classroom discussion. Asks clarifying questions when needed.	Is often "on task" and frequently works until the end of class. Makes occasional contributions to classroom discussion. Occasionally asks clarifying questions when needed.	Is mostly "on task" with some "off-task" behaviors. Works until 5 minutes before the end of class and then exhibits "off-task" behaviors the remaining time. Seldom asks clarifying questions.	Is frequently "off task" and works only as long as teacher is involved. Lack of engagement in classroom discussion. Does not ask clarifying questions.
Time management	Independently starts work and paces tasks to ensure project is completed well before due date. Uses assignment book daily to record assignments/appointments. Prioritizes assignments effectively.	Starts work and paces tasks to ensure project is completed on the due date. Uses assignment book often to record assignments/appointments. Often prioritizes assignments effectively.	Procrastinates or completes assignments at the last minute. Sporadic use of assignment book to record assignments/appointments. Occasionally prioritizes assignments effectively.	Does not complete assignments. Rarely uses assignment book to record assignments/appointments. Rarely prioritizes assignments effectively.
Self-control	Raises hand to speak in class, refrains from calling out, interrupting, or making inappropriate comments to teachers or classmates.	Occasionally forgets to raise hand before speaking; occasionally interrupts, or calls out; refrains from inappropriate comments.	Frequently forgets to raise hand before speaking; occasionally interrupts, or calls out; sometimes makes inappropriate comments to teacher or peers.	Lack of self-control is disruptive to the class—high rates of calling out, interrupting, making inappropriate comments to teachers or peers.
Emotional control	Controls emotions, such as frustration, anger, or anxiety even in emotionally charged situations, such as high-stake tests, confrontations with peers, or criticism or complaints by teachers.	Usually able to control emotions; some difficulty in more challenging situations such as high-stake tests, confrontations with peers, or accusations of wrongdoing by teachers.	Manages emotions OK under normal circumstances; easily disturbed in more emotionally charged situations involving either teachers or peers.	Lack of emotional control is disruptive to the class; easily "set off" in situations triggering anger, anxiety, or frustration.

FIGURE 2.2. Executive skills rubric. Adapted from a rubric developed by Rob Thompson, Cape Elizabeth High School, Cape Elizabeth, Maine. Used with permission.

to see how a skill weakness manifests itself and what impact, if any, interventions such as cuing, rehearsal, or external structure may have on the child's behavior.

Only a few tests have been designed specifically to assess the broad array of executive skills as we have defined them here. Below is a list of tests and subtests that can be used to assess individual executive skills, including a description of the task and the skills it is designed to assess.

NEPSY-II

The NEPSY-II (Korkman, Kirk, & Kemp, 2007) is an individually administered battery that includes a number of subtests designed to assess executive skills in children, including inhibition, initiation, planning, cognitive flexibility, working memory, and selective and sustained attention.

Porteus Mazes

This maze tracing task (Porteus, 1959), according to its developer, was designed to investigate "the process of choosing, trying, and rejecting or adopting a very complex maze" (Porteus, 1957, p. 7). To be successful, the person must trace the maze and not enter any blind alley or go through any solid wall.

Trailmaking Tests

These visual–motor tasks (Reitan & Wolfson, 1985) require rapid graphomotor sequencing of numbers and then alternating number–letter patterns on a page. The tests involve visual scanning and attention, motor speed, and cognitive flexibility or the ability to establish and change mental set.

Wisconsin Card Sorting Test

The Wisconsin Card Sorting Test (Heaton, 1981) is a conceptual sorting task that requires the individual to sort cards with four different types and numbers of symbols on them according to one of four stimulus cards. These stimulus cards represent the sorting categories (e.g., color, shape, number). The test is designed to evaluate the individual's ability to establish and shift mental set.

Mesulam Tests of Directed Attention

This is a pencil-and-paper cancellation test (Mesulam, 1985) in which the student is asked to locate target letters in ordered and random letter arrays. Although this is a brief task, it is somewhat tedious. To do well requires sustained attention, planning skills to devise a search strategy, and self-monitoring to evaluate performance and determine when the task is finished.

Conners Continuous Performance Test-II

This is a computerized attention task (Conners, 2000) in which the student watches letters flash on the computer screen and is instructed to press the space bar or the mouse button for every letter except a specific target letter (*X*). The task requires sustained attention and the ability to inhibit a motor response.

Test of Everyday Attention for Children

The Test of Everyday Attention for Children (Manly, Robertson, Anderson, & Nimmo-Smith, 1999) is normed on children from 6 to 15 years and comprises nine subtests that measure a variety of attentional skills, including children's ability to attend selectively, sustain attention, divide attention between two tasks, switch attention from one thing to another, and inhibit verbal and motor responses.

Delis–Kaplan Executive Function Scale

This is an individually administered battery of nine tests (Delis, Kaplan, & Kramer, 2000) that assess a range of different executive skills in children and adults, including planning, cognitive flexibility, impulsivity, and problem solving.

Cognitive Assessment System

This individually administered cognitive test (Naglieri & Das, 1997) uses six subtests to determine performance on two scales, Planning and Attention, that involve executive functions. The Planning subtests require strategy use for efficient problem solution. The Attention subtests demand sustained concentration for target detection and avoidance of distractions.

PULLING THE ASSESSMENT PROCESS TOGETHER

Figure 2.3 looks at each executive skill and describes how it might appear during an evaluation, including specific tests or subtests that may capture the skill, which behavior rating scales may tap into the skill, and how the skill might manifest itself in everyday life in the classroom or in the home. Evaluators should look for evidence of the skill deficit in multiple settings or assessment procedures.

We should note, however, that in our clinical practice parents and teachers do not always see the same executive skill deficits nor do they perceive the problem as equally pronounced. This does not mean that the problem is artificial. There are different expectations for behavior at home and at school, and the cues and degree of structure differ in the two environments. For instance, for youngsters with problems with emotional control, being

(text continues on page 29)

Executive skill	How the skill may appear in testing situations	Tests/subtests that may capture this skill[a,b]	Where it might be seen on a behavior rating scale[b]	How it might look in school or in the home[c]
Response inhibition	• Answers questions without thinking. • Gives up quickly on challenging tasks. • Gives a quick answer and then changes it. • Answers question before it's been asked. • Tries to begin task without listening to all the instructions.	Conners Continuous Performance Test-II • Response Speed • Commission Errors • Perseverations NEPSY-II • Inhibition • Statue • Auditory Response Set Delis–Kaplan • Trailmaking • Color Word Interference • Tower • 20 Questions KABC-II • Riddles Stroop Color Word Test Test of Everyday Attention	BRIEF—Inhibit Scale ADHD Rating Scale—Hyperactive/Impulsive subscale Conners Rating Scale, Hyperactivity/Impulsivity subscale Teacher Report Form (Achenbach Scales)—Hyperactive/Impulsive subscale	• Talks without raising hand. • Interrupts. • Talks back. • Makes insensitive comments. • Has difficulty waiting turn. • Has physical contact with peers or siblings. • Can't wait while a parent is on the phone.
Working memory	• Asks to have questions or instructions repeated. • Remembers the last piece of information but loses information that came early in a sequence (or remembers what came early and loses the information at the end). • Pauses while working and needs to be prompted to get back to work.	WISC-IV • Digit Span (especially Digits Backwards) • Number–Letter Memory • Arithmetic • Matrix Reasoning (later items) NEPSY-II • Word List Interference • Geometric Puzzles WRAML2 • Verbal Working Memory • Symbolic Working Memory KABC-II • Rover (remembering all the rules)	BRIEF—Working Memory Scale (look at specific items) Brown ADD Scales—Memory Cluster	• Forgets assignments or parts of assignments. • Forgets to bring materials to or from school. • Forgets to hand in homework. • Loses or misplaces belongings (school books, assignment books, sports equipment, etc.). • Forgets classroom procedures. • Forgets to do chores. • Forgets part or all of verbal directions for tasks or chores.

		• Block Counting • Word Order (especially the interference items) WJ-III • Numbers Reversed • Analysis–Synthesis D-KEFS • Sorting DAS • Recall of Designs • Matrix Reasoning CMS • Dot Location • Sequences Test of Everyday Attention		
Emotional control	• Becomes visibly upset or easily frustrated when tasks or items become challenging. • Displays a range of emotions during testing (silliness, anxiety, discouragement, etc.). • Won't admit he or she doesn't know the answer to a question (waits for examiner to prompt or go on to next question). • May make negative statements while working (e.g., "This is tricky," "I don't think I can do this").	We know of no formal tests or subtests designed to assess emotional control directly.	BRIEF—Emotional Control Scale Brown ADD Scales—Affect Cluster Achenbach Scales—Internalizing and Externalizing Problems, as well as individual scales BASC-II—Internalizing and Externalizing Problems, as well as individual scales	• Has frequent tantrums. • Overreacts to small problems. • Has frequent mood changes. • Becomes overly anxious. • Temper flares quickly. • Slow to recover from disappointments.

(cont.)

FIGURE 2.3. Assessment chart. "Be very careful when interpreting performance on formal tests. Just because a child does well in a structured, formal evaluation does not mean the child displays the same skill level in typical classroom or home situations. Furthermore, subtests tap into a number of skills, so it is not always clear that the child has succeeded or failed on the basis of the presence or absence of a specific executive skill. [b] This is not intended to be a comprehensive list of tests or checklists. It includes the ones we are most familiar with or that are designed specifically for the purpose of assessing the particular executive skill identified. [c] The behaviors in this column will be more or less developed depending on the age of the child. For a fuller description of what skill level is expected at different ages, see *Smart but Scattered* (Dawson & Guare, 2009).

Executive skill	How the skill may appear in testing situations	Tests/subtests that may capture this skill [a, b]	Where it might be seen on a behavior rating scale [b]	How it might look in school or in the home [c]
Sustained attention	• Rushes through or gives up quickly on tedious tasks. • Stops working when an obstacle is encountered. • Asks frequently when the testing will be over. • Is drawn off tasks by little distractions. • Irrelevant talking in the middle of working on a subtest.	Scores on subtests requiring working memory are comparatively lower than scores on other subtests or indexes (e.g., Working Memory Index of WISC-IV or Sequential Index of KABC-II). NEPSY-II • Auditory Attention • Auditory Response Set WISC-IV • Coding Auditory Continuous Performance Test Test of Everyday Attention Letter-cancellation tasks such as the Mesulam Tests of Directed Attention Conners Continuous Performance Test • Omission errors • Variability • Hit RT Block Change • Hit RT ISI Change	BRIEF—Working Memory Scale (look at specific items) Brown ADD Scales—Attention Cluster, Effort Cluster	• Fails to complete work or chores on time. • Stops before work is finished. • Switches frequently between activities, including play activities. • Has difficulty listening to stories read aloud. • Distracted by things happening around him/her when doing seatwork/homework.
Task initiation	Weaknesses with this skill are difficult to assess in a formal way since the evaluator is present to make sure student starts on time. Problems with task initiation may be seen on open-ended writing tasks, but this may reflect problems with flexibility or metacognition rather than task initiation.	See comments at left.	BRIEF—Initiate Scale Brown ADD Scales—Activation Scale	• Needs reminders to get started on classwork, homework, or chores. • When one task is completed, slow to start another one. • Waits for someone else to begin in group activities. • Needs cues to begin over-learned routines.
Planning/ prioritization	The planning required on virtually any standardized measure is very different from the planning skills parents and teachers expect from students. You can catch glimpses of it when you see a child use a systematic strategy to	Rey-Osterrieth Complex Figure Porteus Mazes D-KEFS • Tower Test	BRIEF—Planning/Organization Scale (look at specific items)	• Has difficulty carrying out a long-term project, deciding what needs to happen first, second, etc. • Can't make and follow a timeline for project completion.

	complete a task (such as working block-by-block on the Block Design subtest or beginning with configuration lines on the Rey-Osterrieth Complex Figure). Students who do well on tests purported to measure planning cannot be assumed to have good planning skills for real-life tasks.	NEPSY-II • Clocks WISC-IV • Block Design KABC-II • Rover • Triangles • Pattern Reasoning • Story Completion CAS • Matching Numbers • Planned Codes • Planned Connections WJ-III • Planning DAS • Recall of Designs VMI Bender Gestalt Test	• Doesn't offer useful suggestions for how to complete a task when working on a group project. • Can't organize a group game at recess or with friends at home. • Can't complete tasks in the order of priority or importance. • Can't take notes in lectures that focus on the most important information.
Organization	As with planning, the organizational skills required on any standardized measure is very different from the organizational skills parents and teachers expect from students.	See list of subtests for Planning above.	BRIEF—Planning/Organization Scale (see individual items) and the Organization of Materials Scale	• Has messy desk. • Has messy notebooks, backpacks, etc. • Can't find belongings when asked. • Can't produce an organized piece of writing.
Time management	This, too, is a skill that is difficult to tap in formal assessments. it may show up, in a constricted form, when youngsters are given timed tasks, since they are required to adjust their response speed to fit task instructions.	Any timed task, such as the WISC-IV Coding and Symbol Search subtests or the Fluency or Processing Speed subtests of the WJ-III.	We know of no rating scales for children and youth that assess time management per se.	• Has difficulty completing tasks on time. • Misses deadlines for assignments. • Has difficulty estimating how long it takes to do something. • Can't adjust schedule to fit in new tasks, special events. • Can't complete routines consistently on time.

FIGURE 2.3. (cont.)

Executive skill	How the skill may appear in testing situations	Tests/subtests that may capture this skill[a,b]	Where it might be seen on a behavior rating scale[b]	How it might look in school or in the home[c]
Goal-directed persistence	• Stops working on tasks when they become difficult. • Doesn't say things like, "I'm going to get this one!" while working.	This skill is most evident on tasks that require problem solving and when the problem is a challenging one. Puzzle tasks, such as Block Design and Triangles, as well as multistep tasks, such as more complex math word problems may be good places to look for evidence of this skill.	We know of no rating scales for children and youth that assess this skill. The GEC (Global Executive Composite) and the two Index scores of the BRIEF may capture this skill to some extent.	• Doesn't stick with challenging tasks. • Doesn't return to a task if interrupted. • Can't sustain attention well to tasks that are intrinsically interesting.
Flexibility	• Unable to generate multiple answers to questions. • Adjusts slowly to tasks when the instructions change as the task goes along. • Can't figure out a new approach to completing a task when the first approach doesn't work.	WISC-IV • Picture Concepts • Comprehension (questions eliciting multiple responses) • Matrix Reasoning NEPSY-II • Animal Sorting • Word Generation • Design Fluency DAS • Matrix Reasoning D-KEFS • Sorting • Trailmaking • Verbal Fluency • Design Fluency Wisconsin Card Sorting Test	BRIEF—Shift Scale	• Easily upset by changes in plans, disruptions in routines, etc. • Struggles with open-ended tasks. • Doesn't try multiple approaches to solving problems. • Excessively "rule-bound."
Metacognition	• Shows no evidence of "thinking through" problems—either knows an answer or doesn't. • May not realize he or she doesn't understand directions for tasks. • Not aware that more than one strategy may be necessary. • Doesn't check work.	D-KEFS • Sorting • 20 Questions • Word Context • Proverb Test of Problem Solving (both elementary and secondary school versions) Problems with this skill are more likely to be evident on more complex problem solving subtests, such as puzzle tasks, multistep math word problems.	BRIEF—Monitor Scale	• Asks for help rather than trying to solve a problem on his or her own. • Doesn't notice how others react to his or her behavior. • Doesn't like tasks or games that involve problem solving.

FIGURE 2.3. (cont.)

surrounded by classmates behaving with self-control helps mitigate a child's tendency to display excessive emotion for fear of calling attention to him- or herself in a negative way. At home, these children have no reason to be concerned with embarrassing themselves in front of their peers. Alternatively, some children display more emotion in school than at home because school places them in anxiety-provoking situations, especially if they are prone to performance problems or performance anxiety. Similarly, some children exhibit more executive skill weaknesses at home because the demands for independent functioning are greater. Whereas in school teachers cue students to get started on tasks and to keep working, and distractions are kept to a minimum, at home many children are expected to manage homework by themselves, and they have to make choices between work and much more appealing alternatives, such as playing video games or surfing the Internet.

CONCLUSION

To reiterate what we have stated in this chapter: One of the primary values in formal assessment of executive skills is as a medium for the clinical observation of those skills. Tests provide the examiner with a structured set of skill demands for the child. Careful behavioral observation of the child as he or she attempts to meet those demands can provide valuable information about executive skills (e.g., Is there evidence of planning, organization, ability to sustain attention, impulse control, etc.?). Test scores, in and of themselves, do not provide this information and to expect, therefore, that formal test data alone will yield definitive answers regarding executive skill deficits is a mistake. Scores alone, whether above or below average, do not reliably determine the presence or absence of executive skills. We are not suggesting that test scores be ignored or that they have no value. Rather, we believe that observation of the process by the evaluator informs and validates formal assessment data. In addition, we have noted that the presence of the evaluator and the structure of the situation diminish the executive skill demands on the child. Hence, the information gathered in formal assessment must be judged against the child's performance in everyday situations if the evaluation is to have validity.

Finally, at the conclusion of the assessment process, the evaluator should be able to identify specific executive skill weaknesses interfering with a child's ability to manage school-related tasks, home responsibilities, social situations, or any combination of these domains of functioning. With the identification of specific skill weaknesses, an intervention plan can be developed. This process is described in the next chapter.

CHAPTER 3

Linking Assessment to Intervention

The goal of assessment is intervention. To meet this goal, the assessment process is designed to gather behavioral information relevant to intervention. It is not enough, however, to be able to describe the behaviors of concern to design an effective intervention. We must also have some understanding of why the behavior occurs. For example, a student might have difficulty completing independent classwork because he or she is distracted by a peer talking or because he or she doesn't know how to do the task (or both). Thus, throughout the assessment process we employ a hypothesis-testing approach. At each step, as information is gathered we formulate hypotheses about the environment and the child's skills that can help explain the behavior observed. By soliciting information from others and by observing the child in the natural environment and in the test environment, we refine our hypotheses and try to confirm or refute them.

This same hypothesis-testing approach can simultaneously lead to potential intervention strategies. For example, in the above example if the teacher has observed increased work completion when he or she is close by or when peers are not talking, the attention–distractibility hypothesis gains credibility. This information then also sets the direction for intervention. If, on the other hand, the "why" of this student's behavior is not clear, as part of our hypothesis testing we might ask the teacher to stand close by or relocate the student. The outcome will help to clarify the "why" and the intervention strategy.

Once we have gathered our data and generated our hypotheses, the next stage in the assessment-intervention link is translation of these data into a format and plan for intervention. We have developed a process to help organize and synthesize our assessment information for the purpose of designing interventions targeted to those areas of greatest need, as defined by parents, teachers, or both. This process (also summarized in Table 3.1) includes the following steps:

TABLE 3.1. Steps in Executive Skills Intervention Planning

Step 1: Collect assessment information from a variety of sources.
- Interviews
- Behavior checklists
- Classroom observations
- Work samples
- Formal assessment procedures

Step 2: Review data; list specific problem behaviors and connect them to the most appropriate executive skill domain.

Step 3: Select one executive skill domain for initial intervention and identify a specific behavioral goal (e.g., by soliciting from parents or teachers one or two behaviors, which if increased or decreased would lead to better performance for the student).

Step 4: Design the intervention, incorporating one or more of the following elements:
- Environmental supports or modifications that will be put in place to help support the development of the skill.
- The specific skills the child will be taught and the procedure used to teach them.
- What incentives will be used to help motivate the child to use or practice the skills.

Step 5: Evaluate intervention effectiveness by looking at each intervention component and answering the following questions:
- Was the component put in place?
- Was it effective?
- Does it need to be continued?
- What is the plan for fading this component?

---

1. Collect assessment information from a variety of sources, including interviews, behavior checklists, classroom observations, work samples, and formal assessment procedures. Whenever possible, use naturally occurring data sources.

2. Consider each executive skill in turn and identify areas of need in specific, behavioral terms. If you are not sure under which executive skill a particular behavior should be coded, include it under those that seem most relevant.

3. Determine which executive skill will be targeted for intervention first, and identify a specific behavioral goal. The following question, posed to parents or teacher may be helpful in identifying which behaviors are a priority for intervention: "What are one or two behaviors, which, if they increased or decreased, would lead you to say [student's name] is definitely performing better?" For the intervention to be implemented successfully, having all parties involved (parents, teachers, etc.) agree to the goal will be essential. When defining the behavioral goal, make every effort to use naturally occurring data sources (i.e., statistics or other data already being collected by either the teacher or the school). When this is not possible, consider a more individualized measurement system. Table 3.2 lists examples of each.

4. Design the intervention. Three critical elements must be considered in planning

TABLE 3.2. Outcome Measures

Measure	Relevant executive skill
Naturally occurring data sources	
Percentage homework handed in on time	Task initiation, working memory, sustained attention, time management, goal-directed persistence
Homework accuracy (% items correct)	Working memory, metacognition
Test/quiz grades	Working memory, metacognition
Assignment grades • Writing assignments • Projects • Notebook checks	Working memory, planning, organization, time management, metacognition, goal-directed persistence
Discipline referrals/detentions	Response inhibition, emotional control, flexibility
Tardiness	Time management
Individualized data measurement systems	
Behavior counts (e.g., latency, interval recordings, frequency of response, rate of response, percentage of response)	All of these measures can be adapted to assess any executive skill. See Table 3.3 for examples.
Likert-type scales	
Rubrics	
Coaching goals (e.g., % coaching goals met)	

the intervention: (1) the environmental supports or modifications that will be put in place to help support development of the skill; (2) the specific skills the child will be taught and the procedure used to teach them; and (3) what incentives will be used to help motivate the child to use or practice the skills. These elements are all described in detail in Chapter 4.

5. Evaluate intervention effectiveness. This is done subsequent to putting the interview in place. The first step in evaluating the intervention is to review the behavioral objective and assess whether the objective was achieved. Whether the objective was achieved or not, the next step is to evaluate the individual components of the intervention to determine whether they were implemented effectively. Make plans for continuing, changing, or fading intervention components, depending on the effectiveness of the intervention. This analysis might also lead to the conclusion that the behavioral objective was unrealistic. If this is the case, a new objective should be written and an intervention designed appropriate to the new objective.

DEVELOPING BEHAVIORAL OBJECTIVES AND MEASURING INTERVENTION EFFECTIVENESS

The success of this process hinges on the careful description of the desired outcome of the intervention and the agreement of all parties to this outcome. Identifying target behaviors leads to the development of a behavioral objective. This step will drive the remainder of the process including outcome evaluation criteria. According to Alberto and Troutman (1999, p. 66), there are four components to a behavioral objective. The objective should: (1) identify the learner ("Scott will . . . "); (2) identify the target behavior ("complete his daily assigned homework . . . "); (3) identify the conditions under which the behavior is to be displayed ("between 4:00 and 7:00 P.M. with no more than two adult verbal prompts . . . "); and (4) identify criteria for acceptable performance ("for 90% of the assignments given during a marking period"). A target behavior is one that is observable and agreed upon by different staff (and parents where applicable). For example, on the following page we have used the term *meltdown* to describe a behavior. We assume that additional descriptors (e.g., "drops to the floor and cries") would be needed for that term to be operationalized.

Table 3.3 provides examples of behavioral objectives (along with a more detailed description of the data collection procedure) for each executive skill. We selected target behaviors that are frequently a source of concern to classroom teachers. We have identified how progress will be measured, but with most of the objectives we have not identified who will monitor progress. In some cases, the classroom teacher is the most logical person to do this, but it may be more appropriate to have someone else—a paraprofessional, guidance counselor, special education teacher, or school psychologist—be the individual in charge of monitoring progress.

We now offer a case example that illustrates both the assessment process and how that assessment is linked to intervention design. Following a description of the child (named Scott) and the assessment results, we include an "Intervention Design Form" that captures the behaviors of concern and lays out a process for developing appropriate interventions. The example is of a 9-year-old child with multiple executive skill problems. The intervention described is multidimensional in that a single process is used to address many of the needs identified during the assessment process. It does not address all the problems, however. Once this process is successfully in place, other issues such as poor error monitoring can then be addressed.

In the real world not all intervention planning is as detailed or precise as we have described here, nor does it need to be. The guiding principle in designing an intervention should be the least amount of support/training necessary for the student to successfully manage the current problem and similar, related problems as they arise. The latter criterion is important since the goal for the child is not only to solve a specific problem but to transfer and generalize the skill to other problems.

TABLE 3.3. Sample Behavioral Objectives and Measurement Procedures

Executive skill	Sample behavioral objective	How progress will be measured
Response inhibition	In class discussions, student will raise his or her hand and wait to be called on 90% of the time before giving an oral response.	Compute percentage of "hand-raising" responses given over total number of responses given. Student and teacher will graph results weekly.
Working memory	Student will hand in 90% of homework assignments on time.	Compute percentage of homework handed in on time each week; results will be entered in a graphing program and e-mailed to student and his or her parents every Friday.
Emotional control	Student will request "help" or "break" when given an assignment he or she finds difficult or frustrating.	Keep running tally of "meltdowns" (defined behaviorally) during independent work time; graph will be completed weekly and shared with student every Friday.
Sustained attention	Student will complete class assignments within time frame set by teacher 90% of the time.	Count percentage of assignments finished within allotted time; student and teacher will keep daily graph of results.
Task Initiation	Student will start all classroom assignments within 5 minutes of designated start time.	Set kitchen timer at designated start time. When the bell rings, will check in with student to see whether the assignment is begun. Percent assignments started on time will be graphed by student and teacher daily.
Planning/ prioritization	With teacher supervision, student will complete project planning form for every long-term assignment, including a description of steps or subtasks and timelines for each item.	Review project planning form and with student grade quality of planning description using a 1–5 scale (1 = poorly planned with missing elements or unrealistic/unspecified timelines; 5 = well planned, all critical elements defined with precision, complete and realistic timelines); scores will be maintained on a running graph.
Organization	Student will maintain neat desk in the classroom with places allocated for books, notebooks, pencils, etc., and no extraneous materials.	With help from an adult, student will write a list of what a neat desk looks like. Conduct random spot checks at least once a week and together student and teacher will judge how many items on the list are present. Results will be maintained on a running graph.

(cont.)

TABLE 3.3. *(cont.)*

Executive skill	Sample behavioral objective	How progress will be measured
Time management	Student will estimate correctly (to within 10 minutes) how long it takes to complete daily homework assignments and will make and follow a written homework schedule at least four nights per week.	Student will write a daily plan listing all work to be completed, an estimate of how long each task will take, and start and stop times for each task. Coach and student will review previous day's plan every day and rate how well plan was followed using a 1–5 scale (1 = poorly developed plan, poorly executed; 5 = well-developed plan, followed successfully, with accurate time estimates for task completion). Results will be maintained on a running graph.
Goal-directed persistence	With assistance from guidance counselor, student will complete college application process, applying to at least four schools and getting applications in by deadline.	Student and guidance counselor will create a plan for completing college application process, with deadlines for each step in plan. Guidance counselor will track number of cues or reminders needed for student to complete each step in plan; results will be graphed and shared with student on a weekly basis.
Flexibility	Student will use coping strategies to get back on track when he or she meets obstacles in completing class assignments.	Student will complete coping strategies checklist; track percentage of time he or she returns to his or her work within 5 minutes.
Metacognition	Student will use a proofreading checklist for all writing assignments of two or more paragraphs.	Count number of mechanical errors per paragraph for all writing assignments of two or more paragraphs and together with student will keep a running graph of data.

CASE EXAMPLE

To illustrate the assessment process, we now present a brief case example in which a variety of assessment techniques were incorporated. The assessment procedure is described along with the information obtained from that procedure.

Parent Interview/Developmental History Forms

Scott is a 9-year-old child living with his parents and older brother and attending a small private school. Birth history was unremarkable and developmental milestones were within normal limits. There is no significant family or medical history. Scott has attended the same school since preschool, and according to parent reports, teachers noted a tendency to wander around the classroom and to have difficulty initiating activities as early as preschool.

In kindergarten, problems with activity level, concentration, and distractibility were all reported. Parents initiated an evaluation because teachers were reporting continuing problems with task initiation and work completion, as well as concerns about motor restlessness and impulsivity.

At home, Scott's parents describe him as an active child who prefers to be outdoors or on the go. He has difficulty sitting through meals and requires frequent reminders to complete chores and follow morning routines. He is able to engage in both reading and television viewing for long periods of time with no apparent attention problems. Homework completion, however, is problematic both due to difficulty getting started on homework and seeing it through to completion. Scott has friends outside of school with whom he plays regularly. However, his parents note that he has some difficulty interpreting social cues and he seems to have difficulty "fitting into a group." He tends to be literal, overly concrete, and lacks flexibility.

Teacher Interview

In an interview the evaluator conducted with Scott's teachers, they describe him as an active child who has an almost constant need to be "moving or touching someone." Hence, boundary issues with peers arise frequently and require teacher attention and mediation. His impulsivity can extend to his work, resulting in messy papers, broken pens/pencils, and cluttered spaces. Other than fiction reading, he has difficulty with initiation and completion of work, especially if it involves written output. At the same time, they see Scott as a boy who is curious about almost any subject and eager to learn. His teachers feel that if he could better manage his impulsivity and task focus, there would be significant improvements in peer relationships and academics.

Behavior Rating Scales

Scott's parents completed the Child Behavior Checklist (Achenbach, 1991a), placing Scott in the clinical range on the scale as a whole and on the Social Problems and the Attention Problems subscales. They also completed that ADHD Rating Scale—Home Version (DuPaul, Power, Anastopoulos, & Reid, 1998) and placed Scott in the clinical range (i.e., above the 93rd percentile) on both the Inattention and Hyperactive/Impulsive subscales. His teachers placed him in the clinical range on the Externalizing Problems of the Child Behavior Checklist—Teacher Report Form (Achenbach, 1991b) and in the borderline clinical range on the scale as a whole and on the Hyperactivity/Impulsivity subscale. They placed him below the clinical range on the ADHD Rating Scale—School Version (DuPaul et al., 1998). However, on the Comprehensive Behavior Rating Scale for Children (Neeper, Lahey, & Frick, 1990), teachers placed him in the clinical range on the Motoric Hyperactivity and the Oppositional/Conduct Disorders subscales.

Parents and teachers also completed the Behavior Rating Inventory of Executive Function (Gioia et al., 2000). His parents placed him in the clinical range on the total scale, on the Metacognitive Index, and on five of eight subscales (Shift, Initiate, Working Memory,

Plan/Organize, Monitor). His teachers placed him in the clinical range on the scale as a whole, on both the Behavior Regulation Index and the Metacognitive Index and all eight subscales (Inhibit, Emotional Control, and Organization of Materials, in addition to those the parents reported).

Taken as a whole, parents and teachers both reported significant executive skills weaknesses. Parents also reported significant attention problems and social problems, but these dimensions were rated as less problematic by teachers, other than problems with task initiation and work completion. Teachers, however, reported higher levels of acting out or externalizing behaviors, perhaps associated with impulsivity and overactivity.

Behavioral Observations

Scott was observed in his classroom during two periods, one involving independent math work and the other a teacher-led discussion with students sitting in a circle. Percentage of time on task was assessed during the 15-minute independent period. In comparison to a male peer judged by the teacher to have average attention, Scott was on task 35% of the time versus 75% for the other boy. In addition to moving around frequently, Scott intermittently made random, low-level sounds. During the teacher-led activity, frequency of physical contact with nearby peers (touching, bumping, laying against them) was measured using an interval recording technique. Scott was in physical contact with other students during 55% of the intervals in comparison to 10% for a matched peer.

During the evaluation session, Scott presented as initially quiet and serious, but he became more talkative as the session went along. He tended to respond quickly to questions, his initial answers often being both impulsive and incorrect. Careless mistakes due to inattention were observed, particularly on visual tasks, and he failed to check his work for accuracy.

Formal Assessment Results

Both as a device for facilitating behavioral observations and because his parents were interested in obtaining information about Scott's learning style, cognitive, memory, and attention tasks were administered. Scott placed in the above-average range on the WISC-III (Wechsler, 1991), with verbal skills falling in the superior range and nonverbal performance skills falling in the average to above-average range. Long-term memory for verbal information was particularly strong. On visual tasks, inattention to detail affected performance on some tasks, particularly those where there was no easy way to check his work for accuracy (e.g., Picture Completion, Picture Arrangement).

Scott's performance on the subtests comprising the Memory Screening Index of the Wide Range Assessment of Memory and Learning (Sheslow & Adams, 1990) fell in the above-average to well-above-average range for the most part, but he was weaker on the Digit Span subtest of the WISC-III, considered to be a measure of working memory. On this measure, he was inconsistent in his recall of numbers in both forward and backward sequences, scoring at the low end of the average range.

Scott was administered two attention tasks. On the Mesulam Tests of Directed Attention (Mesulam, 1985), a letter-cancellation task, he was asked to locate target letters in ordered and random letter arrays. Although he missed only 4 of 60 targets on the ordered array, he missed 21 of 60 targets on the random array. He spent an equal amount of time on each array, but whereas he was able to employ a systematic search strategy on the ordered array (i.e., going row by row), the random array did not lend itself to this kind of strategy. In the absence of such a search strategy, it appeared that Scott did not know how to evaluate when he was done with the task; thus he missed significantly more target letters. On a computerized attention task, Conners' Continuous Performance Test (Conners, 2000), Scott's response speed was atypically fast, suggestive of impulsivity, but he was able to sustain attention to the 15-minute task without apparent difficulty.

Conclusions

Test results indicate a bright youngster with exceptional verbal skills. The cognitive profile of significantly stronger verbal than nonverbal/visual skills suggests Scott may have some characteristics associated with a nonverbal learning disability, such as the cognitive rigidity his parents describe as well as difficulty reading social cues. Both verbal and visual memory skills are strong, but working memory is more problematic. Some attention problems were seen on clinic tasks. Both parents and teachers report significant problems with impulsivity and activity level, while parents also report significant problems with inattention, including distractibility, daydreaming, and difficulty concentrating. The greatest impediments to social–emotional adjustment and to academic performance at the present time appear to be related to weak executive skills, including problems with behavioral regulation (response inhibition, flexibility) as well as problems with task initiation, working memory, and sustained attention.

Recommendations

Scott has a number of executive skill weaknesses that warrant interventions. Priorities need to be set targeting those deficit areas that are having the biggest negative impact at the present time. Since both his parents and his teachers are primarily concerned with Scott's behavior and performance at school, designing interventions for this setting is most appropriate. Targeting impulsivity and work completion would address the most pressing needs. Strategies should include environmental modifications, a behavior plan built around an incentive system, and teaching specific skills to improve sustained attention and task completion. An intervention to address homework issues would also be warranted. Figure 3.1 depicts how the assessment data are linked to interventions. An intervention to address work completion in school is presented in greatest detail, beginning with problem definition and ending with an assessment of how the intervention worked. (See Form 3.1 on p. 187 in the Appendix for a reproducible version.) Figure 3.2 depicts the intervention design phase for two additional behavioral objectives.

(text resumes on page 45)

Student Name: *Scott*   Date: *10/4/08*

I. Data Sources—check all that apply

✓	Parent Interview	✓	Parent Checklists	✓	Classroom Observation
✓	Teacher Interview	✓	Teacher Checklists		Work Samples
	Student Interview		Student Checklists	✓	Formal Assessment

II. Areas of Need—fill in applicable sections

Response Inhibition (RI): The capacity to think before acting

Specific problem behaviors (e.g., talks out in class; interrupts; says things without thinking)

   1.

   2.

   3.

Working Memory (WM): The ability to hold information in memory while performing complex tasks

Specific problem behaviors (e.g., forgets directions; leaves homework at home; can't do mental arithmetic)

   1. *Forgets to do homework unless prompted.*

   2.

   3.

Emotional Control (EC): The ability to manage emotions in order to achieve goals, complete tasks, or control or direct behavior

Specific problem behaviors (e.g., "freezes" on tests; gets frustrated when makes mistakes; stops trying in the face of challenge)

   1.

   2.

   3.

Sustained Attention (SA): The capacity to maintain attention to a situation or task in spite of distractibility, fatigue, or boredom

Specific problem behaviors (e.g., fails to complete classwork on time; stops work before finishing)

   1.

   2.

   3.

Task Initiation (TI): The ability to begin projects without undue procrastination, in an efficient or timely fashion

Specific problem behaviors (e.g., needs cues to start work; puts off long-term assignments)

   1. *Starts tasks at last minute.*

   2.

   3.

(cont.)

FIGURE 3.1. Executive skills: Planning interventions.

Planning/Prioritization (P): The ability to create a roadmap to reach a goal or to complete a task

Specific problem behaviors (e.g., doesn't know where to start an assignment; can't develop a timeline for long-term assignments)

    1.

    2.

    3.

Organization (O): The ability to create and maintain systems to keep track of information or materials

Specific problem behaviors (e.g., doesn't write down assignments; loses books or papers)

    1.

    2.

    3.

Time Management (TM): The capacity to estimate how much time one has, how to allocate it, and how to stay within time limits and deadlines

Specific problem behaviors (e.g., doesn't work efficiently; can't estimate how long it takes to do something)

    1.

    2.

    3.

Goal-Directed Persistence (GDP): The capacity to have a goal, follow through to the completion of the goal, and not be put off by or distracted by competing interests

Specific problem behaviors (e.g., doesn't see connection between homework and long-term goals; doesn't follow through to achieve stated goals)

    1.

    2.

    3.

Flexibility (F): The ability to revise plans in the face of obstacles, setbacks, new information, or mistakes; it relates to an adaptability to changing conditions

Specific problem behaviors (e.g., gets stuck on one problem-solving strategy; gets upset by unexpected changes to schedule or plans)

    1.

    2.

    3.

Metacognition (M): The ability to stand back and take a bird's-eye view of oneself in a situation; the ability to self-monitor and self-evaluate

Specific problem behaviors (e.g., doesn't have effective study strategies; difficulty catching or correcting mistakes)

    1. *Makes mistakes; doesn't check work.*

    2.

    3.

(cont.)

FIGURE 3.1. *(cont.)*

III. Establish Goal Behavior—select specific skill to work on

GOAL BEHAVIOR 1

Target Executive Skill: *Working memory, task initiation*

Specific Behavioral Objective: *Scott will write and follow a daily classwork schedule, as demonstrated by* *completing 90% of daily assigned tasks with no more than two adult verbal prompts.*

IV. Design Intervention

What environmental supports or modifications will be provided to help reach the target goal?
Presentation of brief tasks; alternate nonpreferred with preferred activities; closed-ended tasks (at least at first).

What specific skills will be taught, who will teach skill, and what procedure will be used to teach the skill(s)?

Skill: *To make and follow a daily classroom work plan.*

Who will teach skill: *Teacher.*

Procedure:
Step 1: The teacher arranges to meet with Scott to explain the process.
Step 2: They decide how often they need to meet and make a plan.
Step 3: Explain the planning template to Scott.
Step 4: Walk Scott through the planning template at the agreed-upon times. —
- *"Let's look at what you have to do."*
- *Make list of the tasks.*
- *Estimate how long it will take to do each task.*
- *Decide on start time for each task.*
- *Decide on breaks or other reinforcers.*
Step 5: Teacher cues start time.
Step 6: Teacher checks in at 10-minute intervals to make sure Scott's following the plan.

What incentives will be used to help motivate the student to use/practice the skill(s)?
Breaks between tasks (with opportunity to move around and/or read for pleasure).
Every other task is a preferred task (e.g., reading).

How will the outcome be measured?
Teacher will calculate percent assignments handed in on time and average number of prompts needed per assignment, using the following tracking form:

> Date: _____
>
> Number of assignments: _____
>
> Number completed on time: _____
>
> Number of prompts required per assignment (circle one):
>
>   1—Three or more prompts
>
>   2—One to two prompts
>
>   3—No prompts

V. Evaluate Intervention

Review date: _____

Was the behavioral objective met?   Yes, completely: ____   Yes, partially: ____   No: ____

(cont.)

FIGURE 3.1. *(cont.)*

Assessment of efficacy of intervention components:

Environmental Supports/Modifications
Were they put in place? Yes.
Were they effective? Yes.
Do they need to be continued? Yes.
Plan for fading supports: Don't fade template, but fade teacher questions as process becomes internalized in working memory and incorporate longer in-class tasks and more advanced assignments.
Skill Instruction
Was the instruction implemented? Yes.
What was the outcome? Scott can make and follow plan without step-by-step instruction.
Does the instruction need to be continued?
Plan for fading instruction: Current instructional sequence already faded.
Incentives
Were incentives used? Yes.
Were they effective? Yes.
Do they need to be continued? Yes.
Plan for fading incentives: Retain incentives but increase work time between breaks.

Date for next review: _____

FIGURE 3.1. *(cont.)*

GOAL BEHAVIOR 2

Target Executive Skill: Response inhibition

Specific Behavioral Objective: Scott will have "safe hands" (will not engage in hugging, pushing, tripping, kicking, punching, pinching, or other forms of unwelcome physical contact) with classmates.

IV. Design Intervention

What environmental supports or modifications will be provided to help reach the target goal?

When working independently, Scott will select a work space greater than an arm's length away from the workspace of another child.

Make sure he is not in proximity to peers with whom physical contact is a high probability (i.e., other children with problems with response inhibition).

Before free-time activities, teacher will cue Scott to use "safe hands."

For any activity requiring physical contact, teacher will define permitted contact for Scott before the activity begins.

What specific skills will be taught, who will teach skill, and what procedure will be used to teach the skill(s)?

Skill: To use safe hands.

Who will teach skill: Teacher.

Procedure:

Step 1: Explain the skill being worked on ("safe hands"). Give alternative things to do with hands (e.g., fidget toys or a directed activity) when he's in situations where problems are likely to arise.
Step 2: Model the skill.
Step 3: Practice the skill, with constructive feedback.
Step 4: Bring in other children to help practice the skill.
Step 5: Cue him to use the skill in classroom and free-time situations.

What incentives will be used to help motivate the student to use/practice the skill(s)?
Verbal feedback; verbal praise.
The alternate activities themselves will be rewarding.
Checks or tokens if necessary.

How Will the outcome be measured?
Teacher will count number of reminders to use safe hands for each activity in which the problem is likely to arise, using the following tracking form:

Date: _____

Number of reminders required per activity (circle one):

1—More than one reminder

2—One reminder

3—No reminders

(cont.)

FIGURE 3.2. Examples of additional interventions targeting Scott's executive skills weaknesses.

GOAL BEHAVIOR 3

Target Executive Skill: <u>Working memory, task initiation</u>

Specific Behavioral Objective: <u>Scott will write and follow a daily homework schedule, as demonstrated by</u>

<u>completing 90% of daily assigned homework with no more than two adult verbal prompts.</u>

_____

IV. Design Intervention

What environmental supports or modifications will be provided to help reach the target goal? Daily Homework Planner Adult prompts to make sure homework plan is made and to cue start time(s)
What specific skills will be taught, who will teach skill, and what procedure will be used to teach the skill(s)? Skill: To make and follow a daily homework plan. Who will teach skill: Parent/Teacher. Procedure: Step 1: Arrange meeting with teacher, parent, and Scott to explain homework process to Scott. Step 2: Decide on a set time to make the daily plan. Step 3: Follow planning process— • "Let's look at what you have for homework." • Make list of homework tasks. • Estimate how long it will take to do each task. • Decide on start time for each task. • Decide on breaks or other reinforcers. Step 4: Parent cues start time.
What incentives will be used to help motivate the student to use/practice the skill(s)? Breaks between tasks. Fun activity to play when homework is finished.

How Will the outcome be measured?
Parents will calculate average number of prompts needed per homework session, using the following tracking form:
 	
        Date: _____
        Number of assignments: _____
        Number completed: _____
        Number of prompts required per homework session (circle one):
            1—Three or more prompts
            2—One to two prompts
            3—No prompts

FIGURE 3.2. *(cont.)*

FITTING EXECUTIVE SKILLS DEVELOPMENT TO RTI

Since writing the first edition of this book, many schools have begun using a RTI process to meet the needs of students with learning and behavioral problems. This is an integrated approach to service delivery that encompasses general and special education, developed to correct some of the shortcomings in traditional special education practice. According to experts (Batsche et al., 2005), RTI can be defined as "the practice of (1) providing high quality instruction/intervention matched to students needs and (2) using learning rate over time and level of performance to (3) make important educational decisions" (p. 3).

To date, RTI has been most widely applied to academic problems and has been used for students identified as having specific learning disabilities. However, the methodology is also increasingly used with students with behavioral challenges as well; thus, it is a versatile approach that can be applied across a broad array of skill deficits, including executive skills.

The key elements of the RTI model include:

- The emphasis on evidence-based instruction and classroom-based intervention.
- The emphasis on early identification and intervention. With RTI, children will not be required to fail before interventions can be implemented.
- The use of progress monitoring, based on objective student performance data, to inform instruction and decision making.
- The use of a problem-solving method to make decisions within a multitiered model. A multitiered model enables services to be deployed based on the severity of student need.

Typically, schools using RTI employ a three-tiered model of service delivery, depicted as a triangle (see Figure 3.3). At the *universal* level (Tier 1) are classroom or schoolwide programs designed to meet the needs of the majority of students. Examples include an evidence-based developmental reading program or a schoolwide positive discipline program. The *targeted* level (Tier 2) is designed to meet the needs of 10–15% of the student

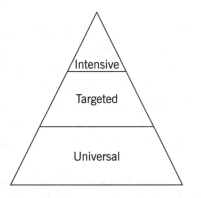

FIGURE 3.3. Three-tiered model.

population for which universal supports are insufficient. Targeted interventions are frequently small-group interventions such as Title I reading groups or social skills groups. For the 1–7% of students with chronic or more severe needs, *intensive* level interventions are required (Tier 3). These are highly individualized programs that deliver specialized instruction, in the case of learning problems, or comprehensive behavior support plans, in the case of behavioral problems.

Our clinical experience has taught us that students with executive skills weaknesses fall along a continuum just as students with other kinds of learning, behavioral, or emotional problems do. At the milder end of the continuum, whole-class interventions are successful. For a student who has trouble remembering to hand in his or her homework, for instance, it may be sufficient to institute a classroomwide homework collection procedure in which students are prompted to place their homework on their desk at the beginning of class and the teacher navigates the room checking off in a rank book the completed assignments.

Students with more pervasive working memory deficits may require a Tier 2 intervention. An example of this might be a small-group coaching arrangement that includes making sure assignment books have been filled in, that students have placed in their backpack everything they need for the night's homework, and that they have made a homework plan that includes attention to both nightly and long-term assignments. Under the guidance of a teacher, students in this kind of coaching group learn to make plans and timelines, develop strategies for remembering everything they have to remember, and make and use checklists to help them keep track of time and materials.

Students who are in danger of failing classes or failing a grade may need a Tier 3 intervention that is more intensive and more highly individualized. At this level, parents, teachers, specialists, paraprofessionals, and guidance counselors may all have a role to play in helping a student acquire the executive skills he or she needs to be successful.

Interventions that are appropriate for each tier will be presented in Chapter 8. For now, Table 3.4 lists the steps that should be followed in assessing the scope of the executive skill problem and designing appropriate interventions.

If the problem the child experiences is fairly discrete, the child's teacher may be able to make a relatively easy adjustment in teaching or classroom management without the need for moving beyond Step 2. Here are some examples of behavioral issues that may be related to executive skill weaknesses that can be handled in this way:

• Sam dawdles over independent seatwork. It takes him a long time to get started, he may engage in avoidance behaviors (sharpening his pencil, going to the bathroom, asking the teacher an unnecessary question), and he often stops in the middle of his work to engage in a conversation with other students sitting at his table. As a result, when the morning is done, Sam's work is not. His teacher feels he is a capable student who likes to get himself off task. She decides to see whether having him stay in from recess after lunch is enough to improve his work completion rate. She puts this consequence in place, and Sam's work completion rate rises to 95%.

• Alicia talks out during morning meeting without raising her hand and would dominate the discussion if allowed. Asking her to raise her hand has not been successful, because if she doesn't get called on right away, she blurts out whatever it was she wanted to say.

TABLE 3.4. Steps in Implementation of RTI for Executive Skills Problems

Step	Assessment process	Intervention level
Step 1:	Parent or teacher raises concerns about behavioral or academic performance that may be related to an executive skills deficit.	
Step 2:	Teacher, with or without assistance from teacher assistance team (TAT) or specialist such as school psychologist, implements an intervention to address the behavior of concern. Collect efficacy data.	Tier 1
Step 3:	If the problem is not solved at Step 2, school psychologist or TAT collects more information regarding the student. At a minimum, a screening that includes broad- and narrow-band assessment of behavioral issues is conducted (e.g., CBCL or BASC-2 and BRIEF), using both parents and teachers as informants. This step may also include parent/teacher/student interviews and classroom observation.	
Step 4:	Problem-solving team meets to design intervention. It may be a more intensive version of classroom-based intervention or it may be a small-group intervention (e.g., assigning student to after-school homework club). Collect efficacy data.	Tier 1 or Tier 2
Step 5:	If progress is inadequate, conduct functional behavioral assessment (FBA) and any other evaluations necessary to better understand the problem. Design multifaceted intervention involving parents, teachers, ancillary support staff, and the student. Collect efficacy data.	Tier 3

Her teacher takes her aside and explains why this is a problem. She suggests they work on "self-control." She explains that she will give Alicia four popsicle sticks at the beginning of circle time. Each time she calls out without raising her hand, she will give her teacher one popsicle stick. If she finishes the morning meeting with at least one stick left, she can choose a sticker. If she has three or four sticks left, she can choose an extra special sticker. Her teacher gives her a sticker book where she can collect her stickers. If she has earned at least four stickers at the end of the week, she gets to take the book home to show her mother. Within a month, Alicia has been able to bring the sticker book home 3 out of 4 weeks. Within 2 months Alicia and the teacher decide together she no longer needs the popsicle sticks or the stickers as reminders.

• Ms. Jacobs, an eighth-grade English teacher, has set up a bin on the table next to her desk and has instructed the class to put their homework in the bin on the way out of class. After trying this for a few weeks, she decides that too many kids are failing to hand in homework, either because they forget or because they didn't do it and they don't see any visible consequence for failing to hand in the work. She decides she needs to make the accountability more apparent and tells the class she is changing her collection procedure. From now on she will stand at the door as students leave and collect the assignments personally. Any students who fail to hand in the assignment will need to wait until the rest of the class has left and then explain why they don't have the homework and what their plan is for getting it to the teacher (preferably by 4:00 that afternoon). With this new procedure, class homework completion rates increase from 60 to 90%.

Notice in each case the intervention is designed to address a single, specific problem, and there are data collection procedures built into the intervention in order to address efficacy. The problem is solved without having to move beyond Step 2 in the RTI implementation process.

For more pervasive or more intractable executive skills weaknesses, Tier 2 or Tier 3 interventions will be required. Guidelines for interventions appropriate for all three tiers are detailed in Chapter 8.

CHAPTER 4

Interventions to Promote Executive Skills

Before we describe interventions to enhance executive skills in children, let's go back and review briefly the developmental nature of these skills. As described in Chapter 1, executive skills are nascent at birth, begin to develop in early infancy, and continue to develop throughout childhood and up to and beyond the end of the second decade of life. Some of the more advanced executive skills do not even begin to emerge until age 6 or so, but the reader will do well to remember that, in early development, any of the skills tend to be rudimentary and imperfect, exhibiting themselves inconsistently. Thus, one cannot assume that if we see a very young child restrain him- or herself from performing an illicit act (e.g., taking an unguarded cookie when told cookies are only for dessert), he or she has the ability to inhibit his or her behavior at all times and under any circumstance.

In the early stages, it is the job of parents and teachers to act as children's frontal lobes. Thus, in effect, executive skills in very young children are first experienced as external to the child, presented as guidelines or limits by parents or other adults in whose charge they are placed. Gradually, children develop and fine-tune these skills, first by mimicking the executive functions of the adults they observe and eventually by making more independent decisions and choices to regulate their own behavior in the absence of adults.

This gives us the first key principle when thinking about how to help children develop executive skills. The developmental progression is from external to internal. When parents or teachers attempt to teach executive skills, they follow this same progression: present them externally first and then—very gradually and potentially over a long time depending on the complexity of the skill being taught and the degree of deficit in the child—fade the instruction, supervision, and cues to the point where the child can apply the skill independently.

A second key principle in developing interventions for children with executive skill deficits also fits this developmental progression from external to internal. Children with

49

underdeveloped executive skills can be supported in one of two ways: (1) by intervening at the level of the environment, or (2) by intervening at the level of the person.

Adults modify the environment by presenting supports, controls, schedules, and other things to reduce the necessity for the child to use executive skills. With a toddler, for instance, we put gates at the head and foot of stairs so the child does not have to decide whether it's safe to climb up or down. We keep food we don't want eaten out of sight or out of reach. We choose clothes appropriate to the weather or the occasion for preschoolers rather than requiring them to make these judgments. And with kindergartners, we're no more likely to send them on a five-step errand than we are to hand them a list of things to do and ask them to read it.

For children with weak executive skills, therefore, the first step is to think about ways to change the environment to adjust to their limitations. While this is often quite effective, the repertoire of interventions cannot stop here; otherwise children would continue to be impaired in their ability to negotiate their world independently. So a second set of interventions involve changing children's skills by teaching them—or motivating them—to develop and use their own executive skills to perform tasks and accomplish goals. When we teach children a procedure to follow to clean their bedrooms, get ready for school in the morning, complete independent classwork, or bring materials home from school, we are giving them a process they can use on their own eventually in the absence of adult cuing or supervision and across different situations.

As children age, the world demands a greater internalization of executive skills. To the extent that children do not require cuing from adults or environmental supports, they are able to move across environments successfully. This ability to move into new environments successfully is important for parents and teachers to understand because (1) it underscores the importance of generalization (i.e., the ability to take something learned in one situation and apply it in another); and (2) it explains why youngsters with severe executive skill deficits are so impaired: They can only operate successfully in settings where the modifications are embedded in the environment rather than presumed to reside within the child.

This chapter expands on these two broad domains—intervening at the level of the environment and intervening at the level of the person. We outline a set of tools that the teacher, parent, or psychologist can draw on to help youngsters with weak executive skills function more effectively. Some of the suggestions we provide are intended for use with individual children, while others are suggestions that can be used with whole classrooms. When teachers can employ structures, routines, and teaching strategies with whole classrooms, all children benefit and an economy of labor is achieved.

STRATEGY 1: INTERVENE AT THE LEVEL OF THE ENVIRONMENT

When we talk about intervening at the level of the environment, we mean changing conditions or situations external to the child to improve executive functioning or to reduce the negative effects of weak executive skills. Changing the environment may include (1) changing the physical or social environment to reduce problems; (2) changing the nature of the tasks we expect children to perform; (3) changing the way cues are provided to prompt the child to perform tasks or behave in a certain way; or (4) changing the way people—particularly parents, teachers, and caregivers—interact with children with executive skill deficits.

Changing the Physical or Social Environment

Modifications for Individual Children

In working with children with executive skills deficits, the first step is to survey the physical and social environment in which the child is placed and determine if there are impediments to smooth executive functioning that can be removed or, conversely, if there are things that can be added to the environment to enhance functioning. Let's take a child with difficulty sustaining attention by way of example. In a classroom environment, just where that child sits in the classroom can have a significant effect on his or her ability to attend. Children who sit in the back of the classroom, next to a window or an open door, or near their friends or talkative students are likely to have a much more difficult time sustaining attention than are children sitting near the teacher or away from competing distractions. Another example of environmental modification would be to place a child with weak time management or planning/organizational skills with a classroom teacher who's highly structured and adept at helping children plan and use their time well. Finally, children who are inflexible, have a weak ability to inhibit impulses, or have difficulty regulating their affect, are likely to do better in social environments in which the number of children with whom they have to interact is reduced and the degree of adult supervision is increased.

Whole-Classroom Modifications

The physical layout of the classroom can support effective executive skills development in a number of ways. We have learned from working with preschool teachers that children are better able to control impulsivity if the classroom does not provide long, wide-open spaces that invite running. Similarly, designing classrooms so that teachers have an unobstructed view of all students also encourages self-control. Teachers should also give some thought to where materials are kept, where children are expected to hand in homework assignments, and other ways of organizing the classroom to encourage organizational skills in students as well as to reduce working memory demands. With respect to modifying the social environment, good teachers give some thought to how they group all the students in their class and where they seat them to promote attention to task and reduce conflicts resulting from placing children with poor impulse control or emotional control within the same vicinity of each other.

At the middle and high school levels, where cooperative learning and group work are integrated into instruction on a regular basis, we urge teachers to take into account students' executive skill strengths and weaknesses when forming learning groups. The student version of the ESQ, found in the Appendix, can be used for this purpose. We have had success at the college level by having students identify their own strongest executive skills and then assigning them to learning teams based on their strengths, so that, as much as possible, each group has students with a variety of executive skill strengths. We have no reason to believe that this same approach won't work at the middle and high school levels as well.

Changing the Nature of the Task

Modifications for Individual Children

With regard to changing the nature of the tasks we expect children to perform, there are a variety of modifications that can be built into tasks to reduce problems. Ways to do this for individual children include:

- *Make the task shorter*, either by reducing the amount of work required or breaking it into pieces with breaks built in along the way. For children with short attention spans, our rule of thumb is that at the beginning of the task, the end of the task is in sight.
- *Make the steps more explicit.* The assignment *Write a paragraph about* . . . , may work for some children, but for those with executive skill deficits, additional structure and guidance will be necessary. This might include spelling out the steps to analyze and solve math word problems, providing "cheat sheets" or templates.
- *Make the task closed ended.* Open-ended tasks can be overwhelming for youngsters with executive skill deficits. They require too much planning, too many choices, or simply too much time to complete. Ways to make tasks closed ended include using fill-in-the-blank or true/false tests rather than essay tests, providing word banks for fill-in-the-blank tests, or allowing children to practice spelling words with magnetic letters rather than using them in sentences.
- *Build in variety or choice* with respect to the tasks to be done or the order in which the tasks are to be done. Have the child suggest ways to alter tasks to make them more interesting or more manageable, or let the child have some say about the order in which the day's work will be completed. This can apply both at home and at school. Teachers might sit down with children at the beginning of the school day to make a daily schedule. Parents, too, often make a homework or chores schedule that gives the child choices.

Academic tasks need to be modified so that the type and/or level of executive skill demand does not exceed the skills of the student. A general rule of thumb regarding task modification is that the student should be able to complete the task successfully without the assistance of an adult at least 75% of the time. Modifications needed to achieve this percentage are less likely to relate to change in content than to change in format (e.g., length, types of directions, mode of response).

Whole-Classroom Modifications

When we think about whole-class modifications in the tasks we expect children to perform, we are in many ways talking about the essence of differentiated instruction. As defined by

Tomlinson (1999) differentiated instruction is based on the premise that all students have unique learning profiles. Tomlinson says, "In differentiated classrooms, teachers provide specific ways for each individual to learn as deeply as possible and as quickly as possible, without assuming one student's road map for learning is identical to anyone else's" (1999, p. 2). Differentiation is achieved through the use of flexible grouping, ongoing assessment and adjustment, and the use of tasks differentiated by content, process, and product according to the individual student's readiness, interests, and learning profile. We would argue that students' learning profiles should include a description of their executive skill strengths and weaknesses and that these should be taken into account when establishing learning goals and processes.

A key element of differentiated instruction involves connecting the skills to be taught with the individual interests of students. This element supports the growth of executive skills as well, since youngsters tend to employ executive skills more effectively in pursuit of goals they set for themselves rather than goals that others set for them (ask any parent of a child who saves up money for a desperately wanted video game when he or she has never shown any inclination to set money aside before).

As examples of how differentiated instruction can support students with weak executive skills, there are likely groups of students in every class who would benefit from task modifications such as the following:

• Students with poor organizational skills benefit from being given master copies of lecture notes to ensure they have the critical information they will need when studying for tests or completing assignments based on lecture material.

• Students with poor planning skills benefit from having long-term assignments broken down into subtasks with timelines and due dates attached to each subtask.

• Students with weak metacognitive skills may need more "scaffolding" to understand concepts and tasks. Scaffolding is "whatever kind of assistance is needed for any student to move from prior knowledge and skill to the next level of knowledge and skill" (Tomlinson, 2001, p. 22). Scaffolding may include reteaching or extended teaching, modeling, teaching through multiple modes, peer tutoring, the use of manipulatives, or the use of organizers and study guides.

• Students with a number of weak executive skills benefit from being given *scoring rubrics* that define exactly what is to be included in class assignments. For students with weak working memory, it is not enough to give them the scoring rubric. The scoring rubric should be written as a checklist and they should be asked to complete the checklist as part of the assignment. Some students will need the teacher to go through the checklist with them before they hand in the assignment to make sure they have not forgotten anything.

• Since there is generally more than one child in each class who requires the kinds of task modifications described above as interventions for individual children, the astute teacher will create a "bank" of modified assignments or a catalog of methods for modifying assignments so that individual children can be more easily plugged into the most appropriate modifications.

Changing the Way Cues Are Provided

Modifications for Individual Children

Another way to alter the environment for children with weak executive skills is to build in cues to remind them of the task to be done or the behavior to be performed. Table 4.1 gives examples of such cues. Students with weak working memory will need cues and reminders, particularly about long-term assignments, but they may even need cues (and monitoring) to make sure they write down assignments in their assignment books and pack in their backpacks everything that needs to go home at the end of the day.

Whole-Classroom Modifications

We suspect that in classrooms where teachers routinely build in reminders in a variety of formats for important tasks or deadlines, a greater percentage of students hand in a greater

---

TABLE 4.1. Examples of Cues to Prompt Behavior

- *Verbal prompts or reminders.* A teacher might say, "Children coming to the reading group should bring with them the reading book, their workbook, and a pencil." Or a parent might say before a child leaves the house in the morning, "Did you remember to pack your lunch, your gym clothes, and the field trip permission form I signed?"
- *Visual cues.* These can be any kind of posted reminder. Many teachers post the class rules in prominent places in the classroom. The best teachers review those rules regularly, particularly in the beginning of the school year, to help the class remember them.
- *Schedules.* Create a schedule for the child, either for a specific event or for a block of time, such as across a morning or across a school day. For younger children, picture schedules are appropriate; lists or calendar schedules are appropriate for older children. Schedules create an organizational framework and predictability for the child, with the expectation that the schedule will eventually become internalized.
- *Lists.* The content of lists may be things to be remembered (e.g., what to take home from school at the end of the day) or steps to be followed (e.g., how to save a computer file). Children with executive skill deficits are often reluctant to do so (it's too effortful, takes too much time, or they're very sure they'll remember without having to write down anything). These children need to be encouraged or required to make lists, and, in the beginning, it's often helpful if someone else makes the list for them and then with them. They may also need secondary cuing systems (i.e., cues to remind them to look at their lists).
- *Audiotaped cues.* One example of an audio cue is a commercially available self-monitoring audiotape designed for children who have difficulty sustaining attention. The tape sounds electronic tones at random intervals, and when the tone sounds, the child is instructed to answer the question, "Was I paying attention?" This can be used with a checklist on which he or she records his or her answer. Another kind of tape cue are reminder tapes, with verbal messages such as reminders to pay attention, work carefully or slowly, check work, and so on.
- *Page systems.* This is particularly appropriate for teenagers since many own cell phones. Parents can text or call children to remind them to perform some task after school, for instance. Many cell phones (such as the iPhone) can be programmed to sound alarms (with verbal reminders) at specific times to alert the youngster of a specific task to be performed.

percentage of assignments on time than in those classrooms where reminders are less consistent and more haphazard. Many teachers post homework assignments and important reminders on the blackboard in the same location and in the same format throughout the year, and students have told us this helps them remember to write down assignments. If teachers cue students to write down assignments, give them time to do this before the class ends (so they are not competing with the rush to get out the door to the next class), and survey the class to make sure every student is writing down the assignment, this increases the chances still further that assignments will be written down and remembered. Many of the cuing systems listed in the table above can be provided for the whole class rather than just individual children. For instance, we have used the "Was I paying attention?" tape in whole classes, and this increased work efficiency for everyone in the class, not just a target child or two.

Initiating class discussions about how students can provide cues and reminders to themselves for important tasks and deadlines is not only an environmental modification, but also begins the transfer from external supports to internal cues that is the long-term goal for all students.

Changing the Way Adults Interact with Students

Modifications for Individual Children

Changing the way adults interact with students with executive skills weaknesses can often help ameliorate the negative impact of weak skills. Particularly with younger children, increasing the level of supervision, support, and cuing is the easiest way to impact executive functioning. There are things adults can do before, during, and after a task or problem situation that calls for the use of executive skills both to help students manage the situation successfully and to help them internalize a process so that they can eventually achieve independence. Table 4.2 lists the kinds of roles adults can play.

When adults are used to supervise, support, or cue, we believe this works best when children are involved in the decision-making process and have some role in choosing what role the adult will play and how he or she will play it. This may include having the youngster help decide what cuing system will be used and what incentives will be available to reward the youngster for responding to the cues. This is another way of ensuring a goodness of fit between the youngster and the environment.

Whole-Classroom Modifications

Teachers who understand executive skills and are committed to helping students improve their own executive functioning weave this knowledge into daily classroom instruction. They model the active use of executive skills (e.g., by talking aloud as they solve a problem, make a plan, or figure out how to organize a project), they arrange for practice sessions so the class can rehearse skills such as how to walk in a line without jostling students, how to use "quiet voices" in the lunchroom, or how to listen during story time, and they notice when students are employing newly developed skills, giving them specific praise to rein-

TABLE 4.2. Ways Adults Can Interact with Students to Promote Executive Skills Development

Before a task or problem situation, adults can . . .
- Rehearse with the student what will happen and how the student will handle it.
- Use verbal prompts or reminders to elicit the executive skill ("Remember what we practiced").
- Arrange for other cues, such as lists, schedules, alarms, or text messaging systems.

During a task or problem situation, adults can . . .
- Coach the student to elicit the rehearsed behaviors.
- Remind the student to check his or her list or schedule.
- Monitor the situation to understand better the triggers and other factors that affect the student's ability to use executive skills successfully.

After a task or problem situation, adults can . . .
- Provide positive reinforcement.
- Debrief—talk about what happened, what worked or didn't work, and what might be done differently the next time.
- Consult with others involved in the situation so that they understand what worked or didn't work.

force the practice. They also ask questions to get students to think about how they might use executive skills more effectively to accomplish the kinds of tasks or behaviors expected of them in the classroom or on the playground, or in order to complete homework efficiently.

Table 4.3 lists the kinds of questions teachers might ask or statements they might make to prompt students to develop or use executive skills. Some are intended for use with individual students, while others could be directed at the whole class.

For students who struggle with answering the kinds of open-ended questions included in Table 4.3, it may be necessary to give them choices of possible answers rather than expecting them to come up with ideas on their own. For example, the first step in helping youngsters who are weak in emotional control learn to manage their feelings is to get them to identify the way they react physically, which then signals to them how they are feeling. Rather than asking them, "How does your body feel?" you might give them choices. In the book *A Clinician's Guide to Think Good–Feel Good* (Stallard, 2005) the author provides worksheets that therapists can use with children. The one that addresses anger asks children to "circle any of the changes you notice when you get angry" (p. 124), and gives them choices such as "can't think clearly," "feel hot," "voice gets louder," "feel tense/uptight." In a similar way, when teachers ask children questions to help shape executive skills development, they may need to begin by giving them possible answers to choose from. They may also want to model the kind of thinking they want their students to do (e.g., "I've forgotten how to do this math assignment. What are some things I could do? I could call my teacher, ask a friend, or maybe ask my older brother who had the same math book last year?").

TABLE 4.3. Sample Questions/Statements to Promote Executive Skills Development

Executive skill	Question/statement/prompt
Response inhibition	• "What can you do to keep from losing your cool on the playground?" • "What can you tell yourself while you're in line to keep from touching the child in front of you?" • "Is there something we can give you to hold to help you remember to raise your hand before speaking?" • "Good job keeping your hands to yourself during circle time today!"
Working memory	• "What are some ways you could remember everything you have to bring home at the end of the day?" • "Some of you seem to have trouble remembering to put your homework in your backpack after you've finished it. What's something you could do to help you remember to do that?"
Emotional control	• "We've had some problems with fights and arguments on the playground. What are some ways you can handle this that solve the problem and keep kids out of trouble?" • "Sometimes kids get nervous when they take tests and it makes it hard for them to focus and remember what they studied. What are some things kids could do when that happens?" • "You did a nice job of controlling your temper at lunch today. What helped you do that?"
Sustained attention	• "Sometimes it's hard to keep working on your homework until it's done. What are some ways you could motivate yourself to keep working?" • "A lot of you talk about how hard it is to stay focused on your classwork because of distractions. Let's make a list of distractions and then brainstorm ways to manage them better."
Task initiation	• "It's hard to get started on homework because there are so many other fun things to do at home. Let's think about ways to get ourselves to get the homework out of the way first." • "I like the way you jumped right into your writing assignment. That's been hard for you to do." • "Take out your assignment books. Next to each homework assignment, I want you to write down what time you plan on starting each one."
Planning/ prioritization	• "One reason we assign kids projects is because we want them to learn how to plan. Let's talk about the steps you need to do in order to complete this project. What do you have to do first?" • "Let's make a homework plan. Make a list of the work you have to do and the order in which you plan to do it."
Time management	• "How long do you think it will take you to finish your spelling homework tonight? Write down your guess and then see if you're right." • "Let's talk about how you manage your time at home to fit in all your homework. Let's make lists of 'have-tos' and 'want-tos' and then decide how much time we can spend on each group."

(cont.)

TABLE 4.3. *(cont.)*

Executive skill	Question/statement/prompt
Organization	• "We're going to spend the last 20 minutes of the day cleaning out our desks. Let's make a list of the steps we have to go through to do this." • "We need a system for organizing our science notebooks. What are some sections we need to include?"
Goal-directed persistence	• "I like the way you stuck with that math problem even though it frustrated you." • "Successful people are those who make goals and go for them, even if there are obstacles along the way. What's a goal you might want to work for? Maybe something you want to build or create, or something you want to learn, or something you want to save up money to buy? Let's set a goal for the month and see if we can help you reach your goal."
Flexibility	• "Tell me three things you can do if you start your math homework and realize you can't remember exactly how to do the assignment." • "Let's talk about what you can do if you get stuck on part of this assignment and start feeling frustrated or angry."
Metacognition	• "Good question. How you could find the answer?" • "What can you do to learn the material that will be on the test?" • "Nice job on that math problem. Tell me how you figured out the answer." • "Class, we have a problem. Too many kids are . . . [losing things, forgetting their homework, not asking for help when they don't understand, saying hurtful things, etc.]. What are some things we could do to solve this problem?"

STRATEGY 2: INTERVENE AT THE LEVEL OF THE PERSON

While inadequate adult support and supervision leads to obvious problems, overreliance on adults assuming the role of the child's frontal lobes also has its drawbacks. Although environmental modifications, including adult support, are important tools that can help children with weak executive skills function successfully, the ultimate goal should be to help children develop their own executive skills sufficiently so they can function independently.

When we intervene at the level of the person, the goal, broadly speaking, is to change the child's capacity for using his or her own executive skills. This can be done in one of two ways: (1) by teaching him or her ways to develop or fine-tune executive skills he or she needs, or (2) by motivating him or her to use executive skills he or she has but is reluctant to employ. In our experience, most youngsters who fail to use executive skills do so not because they don't care but because they don't yet have the executive skill. Thus, we generally recommend that parents and teachers assume this is true and begin tackling executive skill development by teaching the desired skills. However, in many cases interventions at the level of the child involve a combination of both these approaches. This is because learning to use executive skills is often difficult for children with weak executive skills and the addition of an incentive makes practicing the new skills more attractive to the child.

Teaching the Skill

Executive skills are many and varied, and instructional strategies will, by necessity, differ depending on the skill being taught, the context in which it will be used, and the age or developmental level of the child. A general process for teaching children executive skills is outlined in Table 4.4.

By way of example, let's apply this process to a common problem situation in the home: the child who does not clean his or her room. For a very young child or for a child with weak executive skills the directive by a parent to "Go clean your room" produces a response in the child that is inadequate to achieving the desired goal. This response may look different in different children. Some children continue on with whatever task they're engaged in, ignoring the parents' request, while others say, "I'll do it later," and then never do it. Still others complain bitterly or throw temper tantrums. Some children may actually go to their bedrooms and begin the task of room cleaning but get distracted or lose interest before the task is done.

So how do parents who want their child to develop more effective executive skills respond? Initially, they become external frontal lobes for their child. In so doing, they perform the following functions:

- They provide a plan, an organizational scheme, and a specific set of directions.
- They monitor performance.
- They provide encouragement, motivation, and feedback about the success of the approach.
- They problem solve when something doesn't work.
- They determine when the task is completed.

In the parents' mind, the problem behavior is *fails to clean room* and the goal behavior is *cleans room* when asked without the need for supervision or prompts along the way to completion. Initially, parents will need to guide their children through the process by using the following kinds of statements or prompts:

"Let's start now."
"Put your trucks in this box."
"Put your dirty clothes in the laundry."
"Put your books on the bookshelf."
"There are two toys under the bed you missed."
"It doesn't look like all those toys will fit in that one box; we'll need to get another box [choose some toys to put in the attic]."
"When you finish, you can play with your friends."
"I know you hate doing this now, but you'll feel so much better when it's done."

TABLE 4.4. Teaching Children Executive Skills

Step 1: Describe the problem behaviors.

Examples of problem behaviors might be starting chores but not finishing them, not following morning routines on school days, forgetting to hand in homework assignments, losing important papers, and so on. Be as specific as possible in describing the problem behaviors—they should be described as behaviors that can be seen or heard. "Complains about chores" or "rushes through homework, making many mistakes" are better descriptors than "has a bad attitude" or "is lazy."

Step 2: Set a goal.

Usually the goal relates directly to the problem behavior. For instance, if not bringing home necessary homework materials is the problem, the goal might be "Mary will bring home from school all necessary materials to complete homework."

Step 3: Establish a procedure or set of steps to reach the goal.

This is usually done best by creating a checklist that outlines the procedure to be followed. See Chapter 5 for examples of checklists that can be used to address a number of common problems associated with executive skill weaknesses in both home and school settings.

Step 4: Supervise the child following the procedure.

In the early stages, the child will need to be walked through the entire process. Steps include (1) reminding the child to begin the procedure; (2) prompting the child to perform each step in the procedure; (3) observing the child as each step is performed; (4) providing feedback to help improve performance; and (5) praising the child as each step is completed successfully and when the entire procedure is finished.

Step 5: Evaluate the process and make changes if necessary.

At this step, the adult continues to monitor the child's performance to identify where the process might be breaking down or where it might be improved. Most commonly, this will involve tightening the process to include more cues or a more refined breakdown of the task into subtasks. When possible, involve the child in the evaluation process to tap into his or her problem-solving skills.

Step 6: Fade the supervision.

Decrease the number of prompts and level of supervision to the point where the child is able to follow the procedure independently. This should be done gradually, for example by (1) prompting the child at each step but leaving the vicinity between steps; (2) getting the child started and making sure he or she finishes but not being present while he or she performs the task; (3) cuing the child to start, to use the checklist to check off as each step is completed, and to report back when done; and (4) prompting the child to "use your checklist" with no additional cues or reminders. Ultimately, the child will either retrieve the checklist on his or her own or even be able to perform the task without the need for a checklist at all.

"There, doesn't that feel great now that you have a clean room? And your work is over for the day!"

After having walked the child through the process many times, parents can begin to reduce the level of support and supervision. They might, for instance, provide the same information without being the direct agent. Ways to do this include creating a list, picture cues, an audiotape, and the like to remind the child. In this case, the parent might say to the child, "Look at your list." The next step might be to begin to transfer the responsibility to the child by asking a more general question (e.g., "What do you need to do?"). The transfer is complete when the child reaches the point where he or she asks him- or herself, "What do I need to do?" and either refers to the list independently without prompting from the parent or remembers the steps on the list and can perform the task without referring to the list itself.

Let's apply this same process to a classroom activity, for example, getting ready to go home at the end of the day. Table 4.5 outlines the teaching process for teaching a child who has a hard time writing down assignments and making sure all the materials needed get into his or her backpack. An end-of-day routine checklist is provided in Form 5.2.

Teaching Whole-Class Routines

The reader will readily see that it is labor intensive and rather laborious to teach a single child to follow an end-of-day routine. Not only can an economy of scale be achieved when teachers choose to have the whole class follow an end-of-day routine, doing so is in keeping

---

TABLE 4.5. End-of-Day Routine Teaching Procedure

Instructional sequence
- Step 1: Hand checklist to student.
- Step 2: Instruct student to open assignment book and compare what's been written to the assignments listed on the board.
- Step 3: Prompt student to fill in any missing assignments.
- Step 4: Prompt student to write down anything else that needs to go home at bottom of list.
- Step 5: Prompt student to highlight any materials that are needed to complete assignments.
- Step 6: Prompt student to place each item in backpack and to check each off on the list.
- Step 7: Prompt student to ask teacher to sign and date homework checklist.

Fading sequence
- Step 1: Prompt student to begin and cue each step in the process.
- Step 2: Prompt student to begin and ask, "What do you do next?" after each step.
- Step 3: Prompt to begin, tell student to go through the steps; check in periodically and check at end to make sure entire process is followed.
- Step 4: Prompt student to begin and check in when done.
- Step 5: Prompt student to begin; no check in when done.
- Step 6: Student follows entire procedure independently.

with our belief that there are many children in every class who benefit from the prompts built into this kind of routine and teaching the entire class to follow a routine like this instills good habits in all children. Table 4.6 provides an outline and a script to teach the entire class to follow an end-of-the-day routine.

Other Model Teaching Routines

The process described above can be modified to fit a wide variety of situations in which students employ executive skills to accomplish tasks. Many of the daily habits and routines that students with good executive skills follow can be broken down and turned into lists or a set of procedures to be followed. The procedures can be paired with prompting by a teacher, classroom aide, or peer tutor to help children learn to follow and eventually internalize routines that are important for working efficiently and remembering everything that needs to be done. Two additional models that are flexible enough to be applied to multiple executive skills and routines are worth delineating. The first is a process that can be used

---

TABLE 4.6. Teaching a Classwide End-of-Day Routine

Ten minutes before the end of the day, the teacher says:

"Class, put away what you're working on and get out your assignment book. I want you to partner with the student sitting next to you to make sure you have written down all your homework assignments and that you pack in your backpack everything that needs to go home. Listen carefully to what I say:

"Open your assignment book to today's date.

"Compare what you've written down to what's on the blackboard.

"Fill in any missing parts.

"Check your partner's assignment book to make sure it's complete. If you can't read your partner's handwriting, ask your partner to read it to you to make sure he or she can read it.

"For each assignment get the materials that you need and place them in your backpack. Make sure your partner is doing the same thing.

"Place a checkmark next to each assignment as you put the things you need for it in your backpack.

"Look at the blackboard to see if anything else needs to go home today—permission slips, notes to parents, gym clothes . . .

"Put those in your backpack and make sure your partner does the same.

"Sign off on your partner's assignment book and have your partner do the same for you."

While the class is following the routine, the teacher walks around the room making sure everyone is following it and helping out where partners may be having trouble. The teacher should also periodically spot-check the partner to make sure the partner is performing his or her coaching job accurately.

---

to help children manage emotions and impulses. The second involves teaching children to follow scripts (self-talk) to walk their way through situations.

Routines for Managing Impulses and Emotions

Several executive skills—response inhibition, emotional control, and flexibility above all—are all associated with problems involving behavioral excesses. In helping children control these excesses, the goal is to identify the triggers (what provokes the behavior) and to give children alternative, more adaptive ways to respond to the triggers. Here are some examples of how these weak executive skills play out in common situations:

- Maria gets so nervous when she has to make a presentation to the class that she starts shaking and can't remember what she had planned to say. She also gets anxious when taking tests and no matter how hard she studies, her mind goes "blank" and her test scores never show what she has actually learned.
- Tayshon can't keep from blurting out answers to questions during class discussions. He also keeps up a fairly steady conversation when the class is supposed to be quietly working on independent seatwork.
- Malcolm gets very upset every time there is a change of plans, even when the change is due to something beyond the teacher's control (like cold weather preventing the class from having outdoor recess).

Table 4.7 lists a general procedure for helping children manage behavioral excesses in these kinds of situations.

TABLE 4.7. Helping Children Learn to Manage Behavioral Excesses

- Step 1: Help the child identify the "triggers" for the problem behavior. It may be that the behavior of concern happens in a single situation or it may pop up in several different situations.
- Step 2: Determine whether any of the triggers can be eliminated. Technically, this is an environmental modification, but it's a good place to start in understanding the problem behavior and working to reduce it.
- Step 3: Make a list of possible things the child can do instead of the problem behavior (i.e., replacement behaviors). This will vary depending on the nature of the trigger and the problem behavior.
- Step 4: Practice the replacement behaviors, using role playing or simulations. "Let's pretend you. . . . Which strategy do you want to use?"
- Step 5: Begin using the procedure in minor situations (i.e., not ones involving big upsets or major rule infractions).
- Step 6: Move on to situations where more intense behaviors occur.
- Step 7: Connect the use of the procedure to a reward. For best results, use two levels of reward: a "big reward" for never getting to the point where replacement behaviors need to be used and a "small reward" for successfully using one of the agreed-upon replacement behaviors.

The next chapter includes applications of this methodology to more specific behavioral excesses. This same process can be applied in a classroomwide situation when multiple children are exhibiting behavioral excesses in response to trigger situations. For instance, teachers may lead a discussion with the whole class about disruptive behavior on the playground, in the lunchroom, in "specials," or when a substitute teacher is in charge of the class. The class can then practice the appropriate way to behave in those situations.

Using Scripts to Shape the Acquisition of Executive Skills

In Barkley's model of executive skills development, summarized in Chapter 1, internalization of speech becomes a powerful tool for self-regulation. This skill enables children to develop and rehearse rules, solve problems, monitor behavior, and self-instruct. In young children, it's overt: listen to a little girl in the dress-up area of a preschool and you can hear her mimic her mother's instructions: "You have to eat your vegetables before you can have dessert," she may say to the doll sitting in the high chair, and you can see how she is learning to regulate her own behavior. By the time children are in elementary school, this self-talk is less evident, but it can still be harnessed to help children acquire executive skills.

Psychologists and educators have incorporated this notion of self-talk into a number of interventions designed to improve self-regulation and self-management. A commonly used problem-solving model teaches children to ask themselves four questions:

1. "What is my problem?"
2. "What is my plan?"
3. "Am I following my plan?"
4. "How did I do?"

They suggest applying this methodology both to academic problems, such as how to solve a math problem or how to complete a multistep project, and to social problems, such as how to find someone to play with at recess.

Self-talk also forms the centerpiece of cognitive-behavioral therapy. This is based on the premise that how we feel and act in any given situation is a result of what we tell ourselves about that situation. For example, if a student experiences extreme anxiety when taking a test, the self-talk that causes this anxiety might be this: "I'm not sure I studied enough or maybe I didn't study the right material. That means I'm going to fail the test and. . . . [my mom and dad will kill me], [my teacher will think I don't care], [that will bring down my grade for the marking period, affect my GPA, and my chances of getting into the college I want to go to will be shot]," and so on. Cognitive-behavioral therapy teaches the individual to recognize the negative self-talk that causes the bad feelings and to replace it with positive self-talk. For more information about this approach to managing emotional problems, readers are referred to *A Clinician's Guide to Think Good–Feel Good* (Stallard, 2005).

Self-talk has been applied to executive skills development as well. Ylvisaker and Feeney (2002) developed a framework for rehabilitation originally designed for use with youngsters with brain injuries but which more recently (Ylvisaker & Feeney, 2008) they've applied to a broader population of youngsters with executive skill deficits. The basic script involves five steps, which they label Goal–Obstacle–Plan–Do–Review. The steps are depicted as a set of questions and instructions for the child to answer and follow:

- Step 1: "What do you want to accomplish? What will it look like when you're done?"
- Step 2: "This might be hard because. . . . "
- Step 3: "We need a plan. First we'll do this, then this, and so on."
- Step 4: "Do it."
- Step 5: "Review it. How did it work out? How could we make it better?"

Ylvisaker and Feeney have developed a number of variations on this procedure to apply to different situations. Examples of the scripts they've developed include a problem-solving script, a "big deal/little deal" script, a "scary/not scary" script, a "hard/easy" script, and a "ready/not ready" script. The authors also recommend using a coaching metaphor for youngsters who are into sports—for example, using questions like, "What's my game plan?" or statements like, "Call time out."

Examples of self-talk scripts that could be used with children to teach a number of executive skills are presented in Table 4.8. Scripts like these should be highly individualized to meet the specific needs of the child. Some children, for instance, may need a more detailed script. For example, in the first problem situation described in Table 4.8, rather than simply having the child ask, "Did I put all my homework in my backpack?" the script may be altered to read, "Let me get out my homework checklist. Here it is. First it says 'assignment book.' I'll put that in the bag and check it off. Next it says 'spelling workbook.' No, I don't have spelling tonight so that can stay at school. . . . " The script would follow the child all the way through the checklist to make sure nothing gets left out.

Where possible, we recommend having children help write the script. This gives them a chance to participate in the process. It also allows them to choose the words that sound most like them so that when they read the script it feels natural to them. The teacher might read the script back after a first draft is written and ask them to listen carefully to see whether it sounds like something they might say to themselves.

Motivating Children to Use Executive Skills

In addition to teaching children to use executive skills, a second intervention at the level of the child is to motivate children to use executive skills already within their repertoire. Although imposing penalties and negative consequences are often favored by adults to motivate children to change their behavior, we espouse beginning with a positive approach. For children for whom the acquisition of executive skills comes easily, this positive approach may be as simple as providing praise and recognition whenever children use these skills. A parent might say to his or her 5-year-old, for instance, "You remembered to brush your teeth after breakfast without my having to remind you. That's great!" Remembering to notice and respond when children engage in appropriate behaviors (whether executive skills or any other desired behavior) can be a powerful way to shape behavior. Table 4.9 provides guidelines for using praise effectively with children. When that is not enough, however, parents or teachers may find it helpful to use some kind of incentive system to

TABLE 4.8. Sample Self-Talk Scripts

Executive Skill	Problem Situation	Script
Working memory	Forgetting to bring things to school	"The bus is almost here. What do I need to remember to bring to school today?" "Did I put all my homework in my backpack?" "What day is it today? Do I need gym clothes, my trumpet? Anything else special for today? Permission slips? Any projects due today?" "Do I have my lunch?" "Am I doing something after school that I need to bring something for?"
Emotional control	Handling frustration in math	"When I get stuck on a math problem or homework assignment, here are the steps I will follow: "First, I'll read the problem or directions out loud. "I'll ask myself: What is the problem asking me to do? "I'll ask myself if I remember the procedure. "If yes, I'll talk my way through the problem. If I get stuck, I'll follow the plan for what to do if I don't remember the procedure. "If I can't remember the procedure, I'll ask myself how I can find out what procedure I need to use. Here are my choices: see if it's written in the book or in my notes, ask my dad, or call a friend. "I'll decide which one to do first, second, and third. "I'll follow my plan."
Goal-directed persistence	Sticking with a project long enough to get it done	"I have trouble spending enough time on projects to finish them by the deadline. Here's what I will do: "I'll make a project plan that breaks it down into small pieces. "I'll create a timeline—I'll decide when I'll do each piece. "Each night when I begin my homework, I'll look at my project plan and I'll decide when I'm going to start. "I'll set the alarm on my watch to remind me to start on time. "If I want to quit before I've finished that piece, I'll tell myself, 'You can't quit now, you're almost done.' "I'll also think about something I want to do when I finish and use that as the reward—'when I'm done I'll get to play World of Warcraft for half an hour before bed.' "I'll tell myself 'good job' when I follow my plan."

TABLE 4.9. Guidelines for Using Praise Effectively

Effective praise . . .

1. Is delivered immediately after the positive behavior occurs.
2. Specifies the particulars of the accomplishment (e.g., "Thank you for picking up your toys right away after I asked you").
3. Provides information to the child about the value of the accomplishment (e.g., "When you get ready for school quickly, it makes the morning go so smoothly!").
4. Lets the child know that he or she worked hard to accomplish the task (e.g., "I saw you really trying to control your temper!").
5. Orients the child to better appreciate his or her own task-related behavior and thinking about problem-solving (e.g., "I like the way you thought about that and figured out a good solution to the problem").

motivate children to use executive skills. The steps in developing incentive systems are described in Table 4.10.

Figure 4.2 provides an example of how the planning process might work. Figure 4.3 is a sample behavior contract that might be drawn up to address the problem behavior depicted in Figure 4.2. (See Form 4.1, on p. 192 in the Appendix for the materials necessary to design an incentive system and write a behavior contract.)

The Relationship between Effort and Motivation

Some tasks require more effort than others. This is as true for adults as it is for children. Any task you put off—correcting papers, contacting a parent you think doesn't like you, doing lesson plans—is likely deferred to a later time because it feels effortful. Furthermore, what's effortful for one person may feel like the easiest task in the world to another.

There are two kinds of effortful tasks: ones you're not very good at and ones you are capable of doing but just don't like to do. The same applies to children. Although we tend to have a little more understanding and sympathy for children who find some tasks effortful because they're not very good at them, in fact, that second group of tasks is just as challenging and difficult for kids to get through. For both sets of tasks, however, motivating children to make the effort is a key piece of the intervention.

Tasks the child is not very good at are handled by breaking them down into small steps and starting with either the first step and proceeding forward or with the last step and proceeding backward. You don't proceed to the next step until the child has mastered the previous step. Take bed making as an example. Beginning at the end would mean doing the entire task except the last step (putting the pillows on the bed after having put the bedspread in place). Starting at the beginning might mean asking the child simply to straighten the top sheet. The child is praised for doing a good job, and the child's responsibility is restricted to that first step until that step becomes second nature or so easy the child can do it with his or her eyes closed; then you move on to the next step.

It's the second kind of effortful task that tends to irritate teachers because they see a child choosing not to do something that's well within his or her skill level, and they may view the situation as simply a power struggle. Our feeling is that if the task has become a

TABLE 4.10. Designing Incentive Systems

- Steps 1 and 2: Describe the problem behaviors and set a goal.

These are identical to Steps 1 and 2 for teaching the child to use executive skills (see Table 4.4). Both problem and goal behaviors should be described as specifically as possible, usually with a link between the two. As an example, if forgetting to do chores after school is the problem, the goal might be "Joe will complete daily chores without reminders before 4:30 in the afternoon."

- Step 3: Decide on possible rewards and contingencies.

Incentive systems work best when children have a "menu" of rewards to choose from. One of the best ways to do this is a point system in which points can be earned for the goal behaviors and traded in for the reward the child wants to earn. The bigger the reward, the more points the child will need to earn it. The menu should include both larger, more expensive rewards that may take a week or a month to earn, and smaller, inexpensive rewards that can be earned daily. Rewards can include "material" reinforcers (such as favorite foods or small toys) as well as activity rewards (such as the chance to play a game with a parent, teacher, or friend). It may also be necessary to build contingencies into the system—usually the access to a privilege after a task is done (such as the chance to watch a favorite TV show or the chance to talk on the telephone to a friend).

When incentive systems are used in a school setting, it is often beneficial to build in a home component. This is because parents often have available a wider array of reinforcers than are available to teachers. When a coordinated approach is used, a home–school report card is often the vehicle by which teachers communicate to parents how many points the child has earned that day. Situations in which we do not recommend including a home component include (1) when parents, for whatever reason, are unable to maintain the system consistently; (2) when parents insist on negative consequences; or (3) when the child needs a more immediate reward and cannot wait until the end of the school day to earn it.

Once the system is up and running, if you find the child is earning more penalties than rewards, then the program needs to be revised so that the child can be more successful. Usually when this kind of system fails, we think of it as a "design failure" rather than the failure of the child to respond to rewards.

- Step 4: Write a behavior contract.

The contract should say exactly what the child agrees to do and exactly what the parents' or teacher's roles and responsibilities will be. Along with points and rewards, parents or teachers should be sure to praise children for following the contract. It will be important for adults to agree to a contract they can live with: they should avoid penalties they are either unable or unwilling to impose (for instance, if both parents work and are not at home, they cannot monitor whether a child is beginning his or her homework right after school, so an alternative contract may need to be written).

- Step 5: Evaluate the process and make changes if necessary.

Incentive systems may not work the first time. Parents or teachers should expect to try it out and redesign it to work out the kinks. Eventually, once the child is used to doing the behaviors specified in the contract, the contract can be rewritten to work on another problem behavior. As time goes on, children may be willing to drop the use of an incentive system altogether. This is often a long-term goal, however, and adults should be ready to write a new contract if the child slips back to bad habits once a system is dropped.

Incentive Planning Sheet

Problem Behavior
Forgetting to do chores after school

Goal
Complete chores by 4:30 P.M. without reminders

Possible Rewards

Daily	Weekly	Long Term
Extra TV show	*Chance to rent video game*	*Buy video game*
Extra video game time	*Have friend spend night on*	*Buy CD*
Play game with Dad	*weekend*	*Go skiing*
Extra half-hour before bed	*Mom will make favorite dessert*	*Eat out*
	Chance to choose dinner menu	

Possible Contingencies
Can play with friends after school as soon as chores are done
Access to TV/video games after chores are done

FIGURE 4.1. Reminder list: End-of-day routine.

battleground, it's probably gone beyond a simple decision on the part of the child that the task is distasteful. Our advice is if you've fought that battle a couple of times and didn't win, it's best to change the nature of the battle. The goal is then to teach the child to exert effort by getting him or her to override the desire to quit or do anything else that's preferable. The way to do this is to make the first step easy enough so that it doesn't feel particularly hard to the child and to immediately follow that first step with a reward. The reward is there to ensure that there's a pay-off for the child for expending the small amount of effort it takes to complete the first step. You then gradually increase the amount of effort the child has to expend to achieve the reward. This is done either by increasing the task demands or by

Contract

Child agrees to: *complete chores by 4:30 P.M. without verbal reminders.*

To help child reach goal, parents will: *place a chore list on kitchen table before child comes home from school.*

Child will earn: *5 points for each day he or she completes chores without verbal reminders. Points can be traded in for items on the reward menu.*

If child fails to meet agreement, child will: *not earn any points.*

FIGURE 4.2. Sample behavior contract.

increasing the amount of time you expect the child to work before the reward can be earned. The key to success is a very gradual rather than rapid increase in the effort expected.

Of the two kinds of effortful tasks, we may assume that most fall into this second category (the child *can* do it but doesn't want too because it feels too hard). We would caution against making that assumption. Many of the students we work with would rather be seen as *not caring* than *not knowing* (or, more bluntly, they'd rather be seen as *defiant* rather than *stupid*), hence they may try to leave teachers with the impression that they fully understand what they've been asked to do. This becomes increasingly true as students reach middle school, where the judgment of the peer group takes on greater importance. Thus, the first step when a teacher feels a student is avoiding a task because it is perceived as effortful is to ensure he or she truly does understand how to do each step of the assignment.

Using Motivation as a Whole-Class Intervention

Just as teachers can make environmental modifications for an entire class to accommodate for weak executive skills and just as they can develop instructional procedures for teaching specific executive skills that can be used with whole classrooms, so motivation can be geared to groups rather than just individuals. Here are some ways teachers can use motivation and incentives to support executive skill development:

- "Class, for the last 3 weeks, you have been handing in, on average, 75% of the homework assignments. If we can raise that percentage to 90% for the first 3 days this week, then Thursday will be a no-homework night." [Executive skills addressed: sustained attention and working memory] An added bonus for this incentive is that it gives the teacher the opportunity to teach percentages with a real-life application.
- "Class, I've noticed that when we have indoor recess, things get pretty noisy and hectic and I keep having to dim the lights to remind everyone to calm down. If I don't have to dim the lights more than once today, then I'll add an extra 5 minutes to your recess time. What are some things you can do to remember to keep your voices down?" [Executive skills addressed: response inhibition, working memory, metacognition]
- "Lately, I've heard a number of students in the class say unkind things to their classmates. I'm going to start listening for cooperative and encouraging comments. When I hear someone say something positive, I'm going to put a chip in this jar. If the jar is full by Friday, we can have a popcorn party for the last half hour of the day." [Executive skills addressed: response inhibition, emotional control, working memory]

All of these interventions have the effect of bringing the class together to work toward a common goal. If the teacher finds that as these incentives are put in place particular students in the class are having a difficult time meeting the goal, it would make sense to take those students aside and develop a more individualized intervention plan for that student. This might include building in more cues, opportunities for the student to practice the skill in question, or an individualized reward that may be more powerful than a group reward.

HOME–SCHOOL COLLABORATION

Embedded in the notions of environmental support and teaching the child improved executive skills is the assumption that key adults (i.e., parents and teachers) are available and willing to lend their efforts—and frontal lobes—to this task. Experience tells us that this is not always the case. Parents, for example, may have executive skill challenges similar to those of their children, reflecting the proverbial short distance between apple and tree. Or the parent(s) simply may not have the resources or see that the cost of such an effort is exceeded by the benefits. Teachers often already feel overwhelmed by the demands of their jobs, and each new request adds one more straw. They also may see the issue as a motivational deficit rather than a skill deficit and hence frame it as the child's problem to solve. Whatever the reason, the fact remains that a supportive adult is necessary for the success of the intervention. If initial adult support is not available in one or the other setting, we offer the following considerations.

Parental Support Unavailable

When parent support is requested for a school-based executive problem, it is typically around some aspect of homework. Parents may not have the time or organizational skills to help with homework, or conflict between parent and child around this issue may preclude their help. When a parent is unavailable, there are two options. One is to move the homework piece into the school, using study periods and/or an after-school homework club. We also have been able to use after-school child-care programs by providing an incentive to the child for homework completion. A second option is to use a coach (see Chapter 7). This has been quite effective at middle and high school levels where students often resent parent efforts to monitor homework and other school responsibilities.

Teacher Support Unavailable

When a teacher feels that he or she cannot provide the support necessary, there are a few options. If in-class cuing and support is needed, then rather than intervening all day long, one time during the day when the executive skill weakness is most evident can be selected (e.g., circle time, independent work). Another adult such as a school counselor, teacher aide, or speech pathologist could provide the support during this limited time. When carried out in conjunction with a daily incentive system for the child, a skill can be rapidly acquired. With this success, the teacher may be encouraged to provide cuing in other situations to promote generalization, or the adult who provided the original help may come in at a new time. Another option is to use a classmate or an older student as an in-class mentor. One school we work with uses eighth-grade students to help sixth graders with organization and time management. A school counselor or psychologist may also be able to provide a teacher with high- or low-tech solutions (e.g., cuing/signaling devices) to decrease the labor intensity of the support needed. As noted above, coaching with another adult in school also offers an option to support executive skills without adding to the workload of the teacher.

Successful interventions with executive skills are possible, in our experience, even when adult support in one area may not be optimal. Still, chances for success are best when parents and teachers can work collaboratively with the child to first provide and then gradually fade the supports needed to develop executive skills.

SELF-MANAGEMENT/SELF-REGULATION: PULLING IT ALL TOGETHER

Until now, we have focused on what adults can do to modify environments, create instructional strategies, and design motivational systems to support the development of executive skills. But if we're serious about helping students develop these skills, we cannot leave this discussion without focusing on how to involve students not just at the periphery (e.g., by asking their opinion about what cuing strategy might work best for them or having them contribute to the development of a reinforcement menu), but more pervasively, by seeking their input and involvement at every step of the process of intervention design. Self-regulation, after all, is at the heart of executive skills.

Self-management of behavior in classroom settings has been the focus of research since the late 1960s (Fantuzzo & Polite, 1990; Fantuzzo, Rohrbeck, & Azar, 1987), with some impressive results supporting this approach to changing student behavior in the classroom. Fantuzzo and colleagues (1987) identified 11 different elements within self-management interventions where students can be responsible for the management of the intervention. These include (1) selection of target behavior; (2) creation of an operational definition of the target behavior; (3) selection of primary reinforcers; (4) setting the performance goal; (5) administering the prompt to engage in the target behavior; (6) observing the target behavior; (7) recording the occurrence of the target behavior; (8) evaluating whether the performance goal was met; (9) administering secondary reinforcers when the goal is met[1]; (10) administering primary reinforcers when the goal is met; and (11) monitoring occurrence of behavior over time using charts or graphs.

A recent review of the self-management literature (Briesch & Chafouleas, 2009) looked at studies conducted between 1988 and 2008 to determine whether the efficacy of this approach was still supported and to identify which of the 11 elements, were most commonly employed. The good news is that this latest review continued to support self-management as an effective strategy for changing classroom behavior. The not-so-good news is that only one of the 30 studies reviewed employed all 11 elements, and even when the elements were included in the study, more often than not adults were responsible for defining the parameters. Thus, in over 90% of the studies, adults were responsible for selecting and defining the target behaviors and administering both primary and secondary reinforcers. When setting a performance goal was included in the study (this occurred in only about half the studies), 85% of the time adults were responsible for determining the performance criterion.

---

[1] Fantuzzo and colleagues' definitions of primary and secondary reinforcers appear to deviate from the more commonly accepted definitions of these terms. Technically, a primary reinforcer is biologically predetermined to act as a reinforcer, such as food or water. A secondary reinforcer, also called a conditioned reinforcer, is anything that acquires reinforcing properties by being paired with a primary reinforcer, such as a token, points, or money.

Executive skill development is ideally suited to a self-management approach, since the ultimate goal of self-management is independence. As teachers begin to use the teaching routines outlined in this chapter, they may want to use the Executive Skills Self-Management Checklist depicted in Form 4.2 (on p. 194 of the Appendix). It should be understood that while all the elements in this checklist may not be incorporated into every teaching routine or behavioral intervention, the checklist will serve as a reminder to involve the student as much as possible.

To complete this discussion, we think self-management in the context of one particular executive skill, metacognition, deserves special attention. Teachers make a wide array of decisions and choices regarding how they manage their classes and teach their subject matter. Good teachers do this thoughtfully and with an awareness of what research says is effective practice. A substantial body of research on self-regulated learning (e.g., Zimmerman & Schunk, 2001) indicates that academic achievement is heightened when students are actively engaged in the learning process. We believe that if teachers involve students in making the decisions that need to be made about how classrooms are structured, curricula selected, and teaching is conducted, not only are we facilitating self-regulation, we are also providing opportunities for students to use their own metacognitive skills in the service of shaping the environment in which they spend more time than any other (except the home) throughout their formative years.

Many teachers involve students in generating classroom rules; students are also given some say in what they learn (e.g., selecting topics for papers, reports, long-term projects). But what if we looked at virtually every element of classroom and instructional design and asked, "Is there a way to involve students in the decision making involved in classroom and instructional design?" No, we're not returning to that starry-eyed "Summerhill" approach that defined a certain strand of educational philosophy back in the middle of the last century. We recognize that for metacognition to develop, it needs to be guided or facilitated by an "expert" adult (and may need to occur gradually over time, for example, by having the student select from a multiple-choice list prepared by the teacher who has a knowledge of what choices are acceptable). We do believe, however, that there is considerably more opportunity for student involvement than the typical school or classroom allows. Table 4.11 lists a number of dimensions where student involvement could be sought. In the Appendix, we include a questionnaire that we use with students to collect information about interests, learning style, classroom activity preferences, and so on, that can serve as one way to collect input from students that can be used to help promote self-regulated learning. (See Form 4.3 on p. 195.)

TABLE 4.11. Student Involvement in Decision Making to Enhance Executive Skills

Educational component	Suggestions for student involvement
Classroom rules	Ask students to create a list of rules to govern behavior in the classroom. Using a whole-school approach, student input can also be sought regarding rules for behavior in other settings such as hallways, cafeteria, playground, etc.
Curriculum decisions	While curricula may be set by state or local boards of education, where teachers have leeway in deciding what to emphasize, students can be asked their opinions. At a school-wide level, student representatives can be appointed to curriculum committees, students can be asked to complete opinion surveys, or other ways to solicit input from students can be found.
Instructional strategies/ learning activities	Ask students what their preferred learning activities are. When possible, put them in charge of teaching lessons. Have them complete a learning style or interest inventory (see Form 4.3 on p. 195 of the Appendix).
Schedules/routines	Discuss with students the best time of day for different subject matter instruction (elementary level) and how schedules and routines could be adjusted to help students stay alert and focused (e.g., when to take breaks, length of different classroom activities).
Grading policies/course requirements	Involve students in deciding what they need to do to earn grades of A, B, C, etc. Students can also help decide policies regarding late or missing assignments, and can help create scoring rubrics for long-term projects, etc. Where group work or cooperative learning activities contribute to grades, student input can be sought regarding how to grade assignments when some students do more than others.
Rewards/penalties	Involve students in a discussion of what, if any, reinforcers should be used in the classroom, and what penalties are appropriate for misbehavior; train students in conflict resolution to manage disputes between class members.
Homework	Solicit input from students regarding preferred homework assignments. Consider building in choice so that homework selections can match preferred learning style; have students weigh in on rules around homework (e.g., how much, how often, penalties for missing or late assignments).

CHAPTER 5

Specific Teaching Routines to Promote Executive Skills Development

In the course of a school day, there are many opportunities for students to use executive skills. Children need to learn to raise their hands before talking, keep quiet during seatwork time, refrain from making inappropriate or hurtful comments, to handle frustration by asking for help, and to manage emotions when they are criticized or corrected—behaviors that involve executive skills such as response inhibition, flexibility, and emotional control. They need to learn how to organize notebooks, keep track of materials, and keep their desks clean; they need to learn how to plan multistep projects, make sure they write down their assignments and make sure they bring home everything they need at night to do their homework; and they need to learn how to solve problems—both social problems as well as the problems posed by complex work assignments. In so doing they are using executive skills such as working memory, planning, organization, and metacognition.

When teachers use direct instruction to teach students how to get through these common classroom activities, then they are helping them develop habits of mind that are as important as any content curriculum. Furthermore, they can teach these skills and routines in the context of the daily work and daily homework assignments that are already a part of the curriculum.

There are two primary purposes embedded in the use of teaching routines to develop executive skills. First, we present a fairly straightforward set of steps for teaching students to manage problems caused by weak executive skills. The routines included in this chapter generally follow one of the formats outlined in Chapter 4: define the problem situation, outline a set of steps to be followed to resolve the problem, practice the procedure or follow the procedure with cuing and feedback, and gradually fade the supervision.

But if we truly want students to develop the ability to access and deploy their own executive skills *independently*, then we want them to be actively engaged in the process, including the act of defining the problem, generating possible solutions, and thinking about the steps involved in implementing the solution. In other words, we want to engage *their own executive skills*, particularly metacognition, flexibility, planning, and organization. From our perspective, the goal is to help students become good decision makers, which is the essence of mature executive functioning. We expanded on this notion in the section on self-management/self-regulation in Chapter 4, but we add it as a reminder here. As we describe the teaching routines below, we generally identify steps in the process where student input is solicited.

Some additional elements that should be incorporated whenever possible into teaching routines include:

- Be explicit about what is being taught. We can teach an end-of-day routine that involves making sure students write down all their assignments, review the work due the next day as well as deadlines for long-term projects and upcoming tests and quizzes, and place in their backpack all the materials they need to bring home that night. But if we don't tell students that the reason we are teaching this routine is to help them develop strategies for remembering important information as well as ways to improve their planning, organization, and time management skills, then we have missed an opportunity to link the routine to the ultimate goal of having them develop fully functioning executive skills.

- Monitoring performance while the routine is being learned is an essential component of good instruction. This can be very demanding of a teacher's time and attention. This function can be shared with students, however, which reduces the burden on teachers, but also serves as another way to reinforce executive skill development in students. This can be done by assigning a student leader to cue students to follow the routine (with the leadership role being distributed throughout the class on a daily or weekly basis) or using a "buddy" system, where students are paired up to cue and monitor each other as the procedure is followed.

- Evaluate the effectiveness of the teaching routine. This requires teachers to establish criteria for success and to judge the process against the criteria. When using whole-class routines, this can be done by periodically "spot-checking" to determine whether students are following the routine—for example, randomly selecting a different student each day to assess the extent to which the routine is adhered. When teaching routines are used with individual students, the effectiveness of the routine can be measured by the extent to which the outcome is achieved. For instance, if a routine is put in place to help students remember homework, then the percentage of homework handed in on time is a good gauge of whether the routine has been followed successfully.

We have identified a number of common situations that pose a problem in the classroom for children with executive skills weaknesses. In this chapter we offer step-by-step instructions teachers (or paraprofessionals) can use to teach children to manage these problem situations more effectively. Some of these appeared in the book we wrote for parents, *Smart but Scattered* (Dawson & Guare, 2009), but we have adapted them to fit a classroom context.

Many of the routines we describe can be taught either to an individual child or to a whole class. Whenever possible, we recommend incorporating the routine into whole-class instruction since this is less labor-intensive and there is a high likelihood that there are a number of children in every class who would benefit from learning the routines. For each routine, we begin with a description of how to teach it to an individual child, but we follow it with suggestions for how the teaching routine could be adapted for whole-class use and for application at the secondary school level. Below are some general guidelines for adapting routines to younger or older children.

General guidelines for developing instructional routines for young children

- Keep them short.
- Reduce the number of steps involved.
- Use pictures as cues rather than written lists or written instructions.
- Be prepared to provide cues and supervision, and in some cases you'll need to help the child follow the routine, working side by side.

General guidelines for developing instructional routines for older children

- Make them full partners in the design of the routine, the selection of rewards, and the troubleshooting that may be required to improve the routine.
- Be willing to negotiate rather than dictate.
- Whenever possible, use visual cues rather than verbal cues (since these sound a lot like nagging to an older child).

INDEX OF TEACHING ROUTINES

1. GETTING READY TO BEGIN THE DAY

Executive Skills Addressed: *Task Initiation, Sustained Attention, Working Memory*

1. Sit down with the student and make a list of all the things he or she needs to do before the class comes to order. These might include things like hanging up outerwear, getting homework assignments out and ready to be handed in, sharpening pencils, checking the blackboard to see whether there is an assignment that is supposed to be done before class starts, and so on.

2. With input from the student, decide in what order the tasks should be done.

3. Turn the list into a checklist. A sample checklist is provided (see Form 5.1 on p. 197 in the Appendix), but it should be modified to fit the needs of the class.

4. Make multiple copies of the checklist and attach them to a clipboard.

5. Talk with the student about how the process will work from the moment he or she enters the classroom in the morning. Explain that in the beginning, you will cue the student to do each item on the list and that he or she will check off each item as it is completed.

6. Identify what time the whole routine should be finished in order to be ready when it's time for class to start. Write that time on the list, so the student knows when the routine should be completed.

7. Put the system to work. Initially, the student should be cued to begin the first step, monitored while he or she performs that step, prompted to check off the step on the checklist, praised for completing the step, and prompted to go on to the next item on the list. The student should be supervised in this manner each step of the way.

8. Fade the supervision gradually, using the following fading sequence:

- Step 1: Prompt student to begin and cue each step in the process.
- Step 2: Prompt student to begin and ask, "What do you do next?" after each step.
- Step 3: Prompt to begin, tell student to go through the steps, check in periodically, and check at end to make sure the entire process is followed.
- Step 4: Prompt student to begin and check in when done.
- Step 5: Prompt student to begin; no check-in when done.
- Step 6: Student follows entire procedure independently.

Modifications for Whole-Class Use

The same process can be used with a whole class by making it a discussion and asking students to volunteer items to go on the list. A useful part of the discussion might be to talk about whether the list will look the same for everyone in the class or whether everyone in the class should complete the items on the list in the same order. This gives the teacher the chance to reinforce the point that every student is different and some students might have different things they have to do first thing in the morning (e.g., check in with the nurse for medication, or go see another teacher such as the resource room teacher before class starts). Teachers can use this process to help students recognize that lists and checklists help them organize their time and remember everything that has to be done—a handy practice that will serve them well throughout life.

At the implementation phase, teachers may assign a daily leader to take on the role of providing cues to students to make sure they are following the routine. Alternatively, students could be assigned a partner and work in pairs to complete the checklist, reporting back to the teacher or the classroom leader when they have finished the tasks on the list.

Modifications for Secondary-Level Classrooms

Secondary-level teachers may not feel they have to set up the same kind of "getting ready for class" routine that is needed at the elementary level. However, we strongly encourage them to develop a classroom routine around handing in homework. In our experience, homework completion rates are significantly higher in classes where students know that they will be held individually accountable for handing in assignments and where they cannot leave class without explaining to the teacher why they are missing an assignment. Homework completion rates are likely to be much lower when the collection system is haphazard or unmonitored or when students themselves are expected to remember to hand in assignments without cuing from teachers.

2. END-OF-DAY ROUTINE

Executive Skills Addressed: Task Initiation, Sustained Attention, Working Memory, Organization

1. Sit down with the student and make a list of all the things he or she needs to remember to do at the end of the day. This will likely include things like making sure all classwork and homework has been handed in, assignment book has been filled in, student knows what materials have to go home for homework, and student knows what other things might have to go home (e.g., notes to parents, permission slips).

2. Decide in what order the tasks should be done.

3. Turn the list into a checklist. Sample checklists are provided (see Form 5.2 on p. 198 in the Appendix), but they should be modified to fit the needs of the class.

4. Make multiple copies of the checklist and attach them to a clipboard.

5. Talk with the student about how the process will work from the moment the process

begins. Explain that in the beginning, you will cue the student to do each item on the list and that he or she will check off each item as it is completed.

6. Create a checklist that includes everything the student may have to remember to do at the end of the day.

7. Hand checklist to student.

8. Instruct student to open his or her assignment book and compare what's been written to the assignments listed on the blackboard.

9. Prompt student to fill in any missing assignments.

10. Prompt student to write down anything else that needs to go home that day at bottom of list.

11. Prompt student to highlight any materials that are needed to complete assignments.

12. Prompt student to place each item in his or her backpack and to check each item off on the list.

13. Prompt student to ask teacher to sign and date homework checklist.

Modifications for Whole-Class Use

As with the first routine, this same process can be used with the whole class by asking the class to generate a list of tasks that should be included in an end-of-day routine. Once the list is completed, it can be posted on the blackboard (to save paper), but for students who, for a variety of reasons may have difficulty working off the blackboard, individual checklists can be prepared (these can be laminated or placed in plastic sleeves for use with erasable markers so they can be reused each day). During the instructional phase, the teacher should guide the process of completing the checklist, announcing each step and supervising students in completing each step. This role can then be assigned to a student leader. Another option is to pair students so that students sitting next to each other complete the checklist together, monitoring each other to make sure the procedure is followed.

Modifications for Secondary-Level Classrooms

An end-of-class routine will look different at the secondary level, but it is as important as a beginning-of-class routine to increase the likelihood that homework will be completed. We recommend that middle and high school teachers incorporate the following into their classroom routines:

1. Posting homework assignments in a prominent place on the blackboard (the same place every day).

2. Stopping instruction 5 minutes before the end of class to give students time to write down their homework assignments.

3. Prompting students to write down the assignments and monitoring those students who are less likely to do so.

4. Prompting students to make sure all the materials they need to complete assignments are in their backpacks.

5. Cuing students to think about long-term assignments or upcoming tests they need to be working on.

6. Consistently and reliably posting homework assignments on the school website, if this is an option. This is critically important, because this may be the only way parents can monitor assignments.

As the school year progresses, teachers can fade the prompts and cues, but they should be aware of the students in their classes who will continue to need more monitoring and to provide this for them.

3. HOMEWORK COLLECTION ROUTINE

Executive Skill Addressed: Working Memory

We include this in the list of teaching routines primarily to emphasize the importance of establishing homework collection procedures that hold students accountable for getting homework done and handed in on time. Depending on the class, and whether the homework will be reviewed during the class, the actual time and process for homework collection may vary. Components of a homework collection procedure should include:

1. A way of checking off completed homework, so that the teacher knows immediately with each homework assignment which students have completed it and which haven't. This could mean asking students to place their homework on the upper right corner of their desk and having the teacher go around the room checking off in the rank book whether the student has the homework. This role could also be assigned to a "student leader" to save time for the teacher.

2. A consequence for missing homework assignments. We favor asking the student to stay in from recess (at the elementary level) or after school that day (appropriate for both elementary and secondary level) to complete the assignment (unless the missing assignment is produced by the end of the day). For many students who fail to do homework, the threat of a failing grade is less motivating than loss of free time during or after school.

3. A plan for handling students who chronically fail to hand in homework. This might mean referring the student to the school problem-solving team to determine whether a Tier 2 or Tier 3 intervention is warranted (see Chapter 8 for a discussion of Tier 2 and Tier 3 interventions).

4. TEACHING STUDENTS TO MAKE HOMEWORK PLANS

Executive Skills Addressed: Task Initiation, Sustained Attention, Planning, Time Management, Metacognition

1. Explain to the student that making a plan for homework is a good way to learn how to make plans and schedules. Explain that before leaving school at the end of the day, he or she will make a homework plan. (See Form 5.3 on p. 200 in the Appendix).

2. The steps the student should follow:

- Write down all assignments (this can be shorthand, since more detailed directions should be in the student's agenda book or on worksheets).
- Make sure he or she has all the materials needed for each assignment.
- Determine whether he or she will need any help to complete the assignment and who will provide the help.
- Estimate how long each assignment will take.
- Write down when he or she will start each assignment.
- Show the plan to the teacher or aide so that adjustments can be made if needed (e.g., with time estimations).

5. TEACHING STUDENTS HOW TO PAY ATTENTION

Executive Skill Addressed: Sustained Attention

1. Explain that paying attention is a critical skill for doing well in school because information cannot be understood or remembered if it is not attended to in the first place.

2. Ask the student how teachers know when kids are paying attention (eyes on teacher or on the focus of the lesson, raising hands to answer questions, visibly engaged in seatwork, etc.). Talk about what might be acceptable behavior during lectures (e.g., there's some evidence to suggest that doodling or having something to do with one's hands while listening makes it easier to retain information).

3. With the student, develop a brief description of what *paying attention* looks like for him or her.

4. Pick a time of day (or specific class activity) when the student will practice paying attention.

5. Determine how the skill will be monitored during the practice sessions. Some options are

- Teacher or aide sets kitchen timer at random intervals and when the bell rings, student determines whether he or she was attending.
- Use electronic "beep tape" (available from ADD Warehouse) for monitoring attention. This operates on the same principle as the kitchen timer (electronic tones sound at random intervals anywhere from 10 to 90 seconds apart).
- Give student a checklist (see Form 5.4 on p. 201 of the Appendix) and ask him or her to periodically self-monitor and indicate on the checklist whether he or she was attending. If an adult also periodically monitors attention, then student and adult can compare the percentage of time on task by dividing the number of on-task checkmarks by the total number of checkmarks.

6. Begin practice sessions. Remind the student before beginning the session that he or she will be practicing paying attention.

7. Debrief the student after the session to determine how it went. Share observations

or the ratings completed by teacher or aide. Make changes as necessary (e.g., a student may decide that he or she can hold a "fidget ball" and listen at the same time, but if it becomes clear this is not the case, then this will need to be revised).

8. If necessary, have the student set a goal and add a reinforcer to enhance motivation to practice and use the skill.

Modifications for Whole-Class Use

This same process can be used with a whole class. This might include a more extensive class discussion about whether there are individual differences in how students pay attention and whether a strategy that works for one student may not work for another. The same monitoring options and checklist can be used by an entire class rather than a single student. Because many students for whom this teaching routine is appropriate do not like to be singled out, we favor using whole-class instruction to teach this skill. In the typical classroom, there are many students in the class who benefit from the process, so this is a more efficient use of the teacher's time. Setting whole-class goals and the use of reinforcers may enhance the process.

Modifications for Secondary-Level Classrooms

At the secondary level, whole-class instruction in paying attention can follow the same process. It may be necessary to add rules about the use of electronic devices (e.g., cell phones or appropriate use of laptops) to the discussion about what good attending looks like. Adding "pop quizzes" periodically throughout the lecture (e.g., one or two multiple-choice questions about the material covered in the previous 15 minutes) can be used as a way to assess attending. The teacher can ask how many students got the question(s) correct as a way of gauging level of attending (and comprehension of material).

If this teaching routine is used with individual students, the emphasis should be on finding an unobtrusive way for the student to practice the skill. The student could be advised, for instance, to draw two boxes at the top of his or her lecture notes and to put slash marks in the YES or NO box depending on whether he or she is attending. The teacher can check in with the student at the end of class to see how it went.

6. DESK-CLEANING ROUTINE

Executive Skill Taught: *Organization*

The Desk-Cleaning Checklist (Form 5.5 on p. 202 in the Appendix) describes the process for students to follow. The process is the same for individual students and for whole classes. We recommend that desk cleaning be established as a weekly whole-class routine at the elementary level. Since secondary schools do not provide the kinds of desks to students that enable them to store materials, this routine is not appropriate for students at those levels. However, a similar approach might be followed for organizing backpacks and cleaning out lockers. In these cases, the routines would most likely be individual routines, although there may be some value in having a homeroom teacher supervise the whole class in performing these routines at the beginning of the school year. As with all the other routines we presented, this, too, lends itself to a peer-to-peer format, in which students are paired to help each other complete the steps in the process.

7. WRITING A PAPER

Executive Skills Addressed: *Task Initiation, Sustained Attention, Planning, Organization, Time Management, Metacognition*

Students with a variety of executive skill weaknesses struggle with writing papers, and this is one of the most complicated tasks we expect students to do. Use the following steps to help them through the process.

1. Brainstorm topics. If the student has to come up with a topic to write about, the process should begin with brainstorming. The rules of brainstorming are that any idea is accepted and written down in the first stage—the wilder and crazier, the better, because wild and crazy ideas often lead to good, usable ideas. No criticism is allowed at this point. If the student has trouble thinking of ideas on his or her own, the teacher or aide can throw out some ideas of his or her own to "grease the wheels." We recommend that the adult working with the student write down the ideas rather than expecting the student to, since youngsters with weak writing skills often struggle with the act of writing itself. When a reasonable number of ideas have been generated, have the student read the list and circle the most promising ones. The student may know right away what he or she wants to write about. If not, talk about what he or she likes and dislikes about each idea to make it easier to zero in on a good choice.

2. Brainstorm content. Once a topic has been selected, the brainstorming process begins again. Ask the student to "Tell me everything you know or would like to know about this topic." Again, write down any idea or question, the crazier the better at this point.

3. Organize the content. Now look at all the ideas or questions that have been written down. Together with the student, decide whether the material can be grouped together in any way. If the assignment is to do a report on aardvarks, for instance, the information might cluster into categories such as what they look like, where they live, what they eat, who their enemies are, and how they protect themselves. Create topic headings and then write the details under each topic heading. Sometimes it's helpful to use Post-its for this process. During the brainstorming phase, each individual idea or question is written on a separate Post-it. The Post-its can then be organized on a table under topic headings to form an outline of the paper. The paper can then be written (or dictated) from this outline.

4. Write the opening paragraph. This is often the hardest part of the paper to write. The opening paragraph, at its most basic level, describes very succinctly what the paper will be about. For instance, an opening paragraph on a report about aardvarks might read:

This paper is about a strange animal called an aardvark. By the time you finish reading it, you will know what they look like, where they live, what they eat, who their enemies are, and how they protect themselves.

The one other thing that the opening paragraph should try to do is "grab the reader"— give the reader an interesting piece of information to tease his or her curiosity. At the end of the paragraph above, for instance, two more sentences might be added:

The reader will also learn the meaning of the word aardvark and what language it comes from. And if that hasn't grabbed your interest, I will also tell you why the aardvark has a sticky tongue—although you may not want to know this!

Children with writing problems will have trouble writing the opening paragraph by themselves and may need help. Help can be provided by asking general questions, such as "What do you want people to know after they read your paper?" or "Why do you think people might be interested in reading this?" If they need more help than that, they may need a model to work from, for example, an opening paragraph on a topic similar to the one the student is working on, or the paragraph on aardvarks provided here. If the student needs more guided help writing this paragraph, provide it. Then see if he or she can continue without the need for as much support.

5. Write the rest of the paper. To give the student a little more guidance, suggest that the rest of the paper be divided into sections with a heading for each section. Help him or her make a list of the headings and then see if he or she can continue with the writing task alone. If not, continue to provide support until the paper is written. Each paragraph should begin with a main or topic sentence that makes one main point. Following the topic sentence should be three to five sentences that expand or explain the main point. It's helpful to use connecting words to link sentences or paragraphs. Examples of simple linking words are *and, because, also, instead, but, and so.* Examples of more complex linking words are *although, moreover, on the other hand, therefore, as a result, finally, and in conclusion.*

In the early stages of learning to write, children with writing problems need a great deal of help. It should get better with time, especially if each writing session concludes by giving the student some positive feedback about something done well. Note in particular any improvement since the last writing assignment (e.g., "I really like the way you were able to come up with the headings on your own this time, with no help from me.").

Modifications for Whole-Class Use

When using this process with the whole class, the teacher should model the process, thinking aloud as he or she proceeds through the steps. During the brainstorming phases, students should be called upon to contribute material, with the teacher reinforcing the rules of brainstorming as needed (e.g., no criticizing). Students should be given a blank template and instructed to copy down what the teacher writes (for students with writing difficulties, a completed template can be provided as a model) so that when the lesson is over, they have an example of an essay that they can work from for future writing assignments. (See Form 5.6 on p. 203 in the Appendix for a reproducible template.)

Students will need lots of practice to master the skill of essay writing. Pairing students to write essays together following the template is one way to give them this practice before assigning individual essays for homework.

For Students with More Significant Writing Impairments

More modeling, guidance, and support will need to be provided for students with writing disabilities. Furthermore, the process may need to be broken down a good deal more. For students with significant impairments or for students who are highly resistant to the writing process, we recommend the following sequence:

- Step 1: Spend a few minutes (e.g., 5 minutes) daily practicing any kind of writing. Here the goal is to get words down on paper. For many students, just having them write any words they can think of is the place to start. If children have difficulty generating words on their own, give them organizing or retrieval strategies—such as looking around the room and writing down the name of anything they see, or having them write rhyming words by giving them the first word (e.g., *cat, man*). Count the number of words written and keep a graph, challenging them to write a few more words each day.
- Step 2: Give students a picture and have them write down words to describe the picture or have them describe the picture and you write down the words. Use pictures that reflect the child's interests.
- Step 3: Give students a picture and have them write a sentence or two describing the picture.
- Step 4: Have students draw a picture and write sentences describing the picture or telling a story to go along with the picture.
- Step 5: Finally, give students a story starter and have them write for 5 minutes based on the story starter. They may want to choose a story starter or to think up one on their own.

This approach can be very effective when combined with curriculum-based measurement—that is, keeping the time frame constant, counting the number of words written, and graphing the results. The graph should be constructed with the child, and might incorporate small stickers (obtainable at an office supply store) to construct the graph. Watching the graph go up can be very motivating for young children in particular with written production problems.

Additional Resources

Harvey, V. S., & Chickie-Wolfe, L. A. (2007). *Fostering independent learning: Practical strategies to promote student success.*—New York: Guilford Press. This book has a chapter devoted to writing that includes a number of useful checklists and handouts. One handout lists a wide variety of "genre ideas" that reminds teachers that there are a wide variety of forms of writing and going beyond the traditional essay may help stimulate writing in reluctant writers.

Harris, K. R., Graham, S., Mason, L. H., & Friedlander, B. (2008). *Powerful writing strategies for all students.* Baltimore: Brookes.—This book describes the process of Self-Regulated Strategy Development and applies it to the writing process. Packed with helpful lesson plans and handouts, it details explicit strategies for specific writing genres as well as general writing strategies with an overarching goal of developing self-regulated learners. Thus, not only does the book teach writing, but it also helps students learn self-regulation strategies (i.e., executive skills!) such as goals-setting, self-monitoring, self-reinforcement, and self-instruction.

8. LONG-TERM PROJECTS

***Executive Skills Addressed:** Task Initiation, Sustained Attention, Planning, Time Management, Metacognition*

Even more than writing assignments, long-term projects involve many of the more advanced executive skills. For this reason, students in general benefit from teacher support, not only when this kind of assignment is first introduced but to some degree or other throughout their schooling (at least until well into high school). The steps involved teaching students to complete long-term projects are as follows:

1. With the student, look at the description of the assignment to make sure he or she understands what is expected. If the assignment allows the student a choice of topic, topic selection is the first step. Many children have trouble thinking up topics, and if this is the case, then brainstorming topic ideas may need to include providing lots of suggestions, starting with topics that are related to the student's areas of interests.

2. Using the Project-Planning Sheet (Form 5.7 on p. 205 in the Appendix), write down the possible topics. Once three to five have been generated, ask the student what he/she likes and doesn't like about each choice.

3. Help the student make a final selection. In addition to thinking about what topic is of greatest interest, other things to think about in making a final selection are (1) choosing a topic that is neither too broad nor too narrow; (2) how difficult it will be to track down references and resources; and (3) whether there is an interesting "twist" to the topic that will either make it fun to work on or appealing for the teacher.

4. Using the Project-Planning Sheet, decide what materials or resources will be needed, where the student will get them, and when (this last column may be filled in after completing the next step). Possible resources include Internet websites, library books, things that may need to be ordered (e.g., travel brochures), people who might be interviewed, or places to visit (e.g., museums, historical sites). You may need to "walk" the student through the process of tracking down sources (e.g., going to the library or going on the Internet to show how to conduct a search). Also consider any construction or art materials that will be needed if the project involves building something.

5. Using the Project-Planning Sheet, list all the steps that will need to be done to carry out the project and then develop a timeline so the student knows when each step will be

done. It may be helpful at this point to transfer this information onto a monthly calendar that can be placed in the student's binder to make it easier to keep track of what needs to be done and when.

6. Assist the student in following the timeline. Before he or she begins each step, you may want to have a discussion about what exactly is involved in completing the step—this may mean making a list of things to be done for each step. Planning for the next step could be done as each step is completed, so that the student has some idea what's coming next and to make it easier to get the next step started.

Modifications for Whole-Class Use

The same routine can be taught to whole classes. As with the paper-writing routine, students can be paired to complete the Project-Planning Form together. When group projects are assigned, the first step in the project would be to have the group complete the Project-Planning Form. Depending on the kind of project assigned, the form may need to be modified (e.g., by adding a "Person Responsible" column).

Modifications for Secondary-Level Classrooms

Students at all age levels and of all abilities have a tendency to procrastinate. Those with poor planning and time management skills are particularly likely to misjudge what they can accomplish at the last minute, but we think all students benefit from assistance in developing a long-term project plan. We also think firm interim deadlines should be built into the process to support the "habit building" that's required for students to learn to manage this kind of task independently. Teachers can help transfer this skill to students by eventually asking them to develop their own timelines and interim deadlines. When this is done, the timeline should be reviewed individually and the teacher should check back with each student to make sure the project is on schedule. The teacher may want to create a master calendar in which each student's interim deadline is identified so that the teacher can check in with students on the right date. This role could conceivably be assigned to a student monitor, but the role of that person should be carefully specified (e.g., what evidence should the student look for to ensure the deadline is met, what should the student do if the deadline is missed).

9. STUDYING FOR TESTS

Executive Skills Addressed: Task Initiation, Sustained Attention, Planning, Time Management, Metacognition

We see many students who readily admit to us that they rarely study for tests. When we ask them what strategies they use when they do study, they either report a passive study method (such as "I reread my notes," "I scan the text") or they admit that they really don't know how to study. If you ask their teachers, they often say, "The problem is that the student chooses not to study," but are often confident nevertheless that they know how to study if they choose to. As with any other task involving executive skills, we begin from the premise that the student actually doesn't know how to study for tests. We suggest the following process to help students learn how to study for tests. (See Form 5.8 on p. 207 in the Appendix for all the studying tools discussed.)

1. Keep a monthly calendar with the student on which any upcoming tests are written.

2. From 5 days to a week before the test, create a study plan with the student.

3. Using the Study Strategies Menu, have the student decide which strategies he or she wants to use to study for the test. Make sure he or she understands what's involved in each strategy, providing further explanation if necessary (e.g., if the student chooses "Study flash cards," ask him or her to show what the flash cards will look like, giving additional suggestions for flash card design).

4. Have the student make a plan for studying that starts 4 days before the test. Psychological research over many years shows that when new material is learned, distributed practice is more effective than massed practice. In other words, if you plan to spend 2 hours studying for a test, it is better to break down the time into smaller segments (such as 30 minutes a night for 4 nights) than to spend the full 2 hours studying the night before the test. Research also shows that learning is consolidated through sleep, so getting a good night's sleep the night before an exam is more beneficial than "cramming" the night before.

5. For students who have problems with sustained attention, using several strategies each for a short amount of time may be easier than using one strategy for the full study period. You can suggest they set a kitchen timer for the length of time for each strategy, and when the bell rings, the student can move on to the next strategy (unless the student likes the one being used and wants to continue it).

6. After the student takes the test, have him or her complete the posttest evaluation. This builds self-evaluation so that improvements can be made the next time a test comes up.

Modifications for Whole-Class Use

This is a useful skill to teach an entire class. Several components to include when introducing the topic:

1. Talk about the importance of using active study strategies, and explain the research on massed versus distributed practice.

2. Explain that what works for one student may not work for another, and it's important to identify the strategies that work best for each student. Ask students to share the different strategies they use that they find helpful. Be sure to explain that different strategies should be used for different kinds of tests, and that students should select strategies appropriate to the kind of test they will be taking.

3. Let students know that one reason students do poorly on tests is because they don't study long enough. Talk about strategies students can use to motivate themselves to persist

with studying even if they find it "boring." Introduce the concept of self-talk ("What could you say to yourself to keep yourself going?") as well as the notion of self-rewards ("Can you think of a reward you could give yourself when you meet your study goal?"). Let them know that using a variety of study strategies, each for a short period of time, is one way to keep the task from being too tedious.

4. Introduce the Study Plan and clarify any of the strategies that might not be understood by students. Teachers may want to model some of these strategies (e.g., how to highlight notes, make flash cards, quiz oneself), or even better, assign students to small groups, give each group a different strategy, and ask them to prepare a small skit that models the strategy.

5. Have students create their own personalized study plan. If desired, teachers could assign the whole class to use the same strategy as part of their study plan as a way to reinforce a particular study strategy.

Modifications for Secondary-Level Classrooms

Even at the secondary level, a surprising number of students don't know how to study for tests. We recommend using whole-class instruction for this skill as described above.

10. ORGANIZING NOTEBOOKS/HOMEWORK

Executive Skills Addressed: Organization, Task Initiation

1. With input from the student, decide on what needs to be included in the organizational system: A place to keep unfinished homework? A separate place to keep completed homework? A place to keep papers that need to be filed? Notebooks or binders to keep notes, completed assignments, handouts, worksheets, and so on? A sample list can be found in Form 5.9 (on p. 208 in the Appendix).

2. Once you've listed all these elements, decide how best to handle them, one at a time. For example, you and the student might decide on a colored folder system, with a different color for completed assignments, unfinished work, and other papers. Or you might decide to have a separate small three-ring binder for each subject or one large binder to handle all subjects.

3. Make a list of the materials the student needs; these might include a three-hole punch, lined and unlined paper, subject dividers, and small Post-it packages the student might want to use to flag important papers.

4. Ask the student to procure the necessary materials if they are not available at school. It may be necessary to e-mail the student's parents to ensure the materials are obtained.

5. Set up the notebooks and folders, labeling everything clearly.

6. Help the student maintain the system over time using Form 5.9. This generally means a daily check-in that might include having the student take out the folders for completed assignments, unfinished work, and material to be filed. Have the student make a decision about each piece of material and where it should go.

Modifications for Whole-Class Use or for Use in Secondary-Level Classrooms

Teachers often have a preferred way for students to organize the notebooks for the subjects that they teach. When this is the case, directions for organizing notebooks should be provided in writing. This could be a combination of a checklist for setting up the notebook and a scoring rubric that informs students how the notebook will be graded. Commonly, students are graded on whether the notebook contains all required sections, whether headers and/or footers are included, and how well the notebooks are organized (e.g., materials in a logical or numerical sequence or chronological order, and neatness). If this is an important component of the report card grade, then regular notebook checks should be instituted and consequences should be imposed for missing elements or low scores (e.g., a daily or weekly check rather than a biweekly or monthly check).

11. MANAGING OPEN-ENDED TASKS

Executive Skills Addressed: *Emotional Control, Flexibility, Metacognition*

For many students, the most challenging assignment is one that involves an open-ended task. Open-ended tasks are those in which (1) multiple correct answers are possible; (2) there are different ways to achieve the correct answer or desired result; (3) the task itself provides no clear feedback about its completion, leaving it to the student to decide when he or she is done; or (4) the task has no obvious starting point, leaving it to the student to decide what to do first.

Examples of open-ended tasks include:

- Using spelling words in sentences
- Any writing assignment
- Showing several ways to solve a math problem (e.g., "How many different ways can you group 24 items into even-numbered groups?")
- Selecting a strategy to solve a more complex math word problem
- Answering "Why?" questions
- Looking for answers to social studies questions in the text, unless the correct answer is one word or a concrete concept

There are two ways to help students with open-ended tasks:

1. Revise the tasks to make them more closed ended.
2. Teach them how to handle these kinds of tasks.

Since problems handling open-ended tasks are most evident when children do open-ended homework assignments, teachers should be alert to this kind of problem when checking homework or when talking with parents about homework problems.

Ways to make open-ended tasks more closed ended include the following:

1. Talk the student through the task—either help him or her get started or talk about each step in the task and stay with the student while he or she performs each step.

2. Don't ask the student to come up with ideas on his or her own—give him or her choices or narrow the number of choices. Over time, you can fade this modification, for instance, by gradually increasing the number of choices or by encouraging the student to add to the choices you're providing.

3. Give the student "cheat sheets" or procedure lists (e.g., the steps in a math process such as long division).

4. Alter the task to remove the problem-solving demand. For instance, practice spelling words by writing each word 10 times rather than composing sentences or give the student sentences with the spelling words missing.

5. Provide templates for writing assignments. The template itself then can walk the child through the task.

6. Provide ample support in the prewriting phases, in particular, brainstorming ideas for writing assignments and organizing those ideas (see Writing a Paper).

7. Provide scoring rubrics that spell out exactly what is expected for any assignment.

The easiest way to help the student become more adept with open-ended tasks is to walk him or her through the task, using a think-aloud procedure. In other words, model the kinds of thoughts and strategies needed to attack the task. This generally involves providing close guidance and lots of support initially and then gradually fading the support, handing over the planning more and more to the student. For students with significant problems with flexibility, managing open-ended tasks successfully often takes years and thus may require assignment modifications and support for a long time.

12. TEACHING STUDENTS HOW TO TAKE NOTES

Executive Skills Addressed: Organization, Metacognition

1. Solicit from student the reasons note taking is important. If the student has difficulty answering the question, point out that note taking not only enables students to record important information they will need to understand the lecture topic and provides material they can use when studying for tests, but it is also a way to help them pay attention and focus on the class.

2. Ask the student how he or she takes notes now and to assess how useful the method is. Explain that learning is most likely to occur when three things happen: (1) the student is able to absorb the relevant information in a way that's organized appropriately for the material being presented; (2) the student is able to extract the key concepts or main ideas as a way to help in understanding and retaining the factual information presented in a lecture; and (3) the student is able to apply what he or she is learning to prior learning or relate it to personal experiences in order to have a meaningful context within which the new material

can be placed. The more a student can make the information *emotionally* relevant, the more he or she is likely to understand and remember.

3. If the student's current note-taking style does not incorporate these three elements, then explain that you will be teaching the student a couple of different note-taking strategies to try out and decide which one works best.

Note-Taking Strategy 1: Cornell Method

This strategy employs three-column note paper (Form 5.10 is a sample template you can use; see p. 209 in the Appendix) and begins with sequential note taking (writing down what the teacher is saying in the sequence provided) in the center column. As the lecture progresses, the student writes down key concepts and "big ideas" in the left-hand column. Sometimes teachers are direct in saying what those key concepts are, but sometimes students have to listen carefully and draw conclusions on their own. In the right-hand column, the student is instructed to jot down personal reflections, such as a word or two that relates the material to a personal experience, an emotional reaction to what is being said, or a question about the lecture material. The first and third columns can be filled in during the lecture as well as later, when the student reviews the notes from the day's class.

The strategy should be modeled using relevant material from the class in which the note taking will be used. The student may need particular help identifying key concepts or relating the material to personal experiences and can be guided through this process by asking questions (e.g., "Can you think of anything in your life that you could relate this to?" "What's your opinion about this—do you agree or disagree?").

If teachers provide PowerPoint notes to students, they can use a highlighter to highlight key concepts and in the margins can write down personal reactions/questions. This, too, may need to be modeled for some students.

Note-Taking Strategy 2: Concept Mapping

This is a visual strategy in which graphic organizers are employed to link key concepts to details. Concept maps begin with a central topic (e.g., the title of the day's lecture), to which main branches are added to represent the main subdivisions of the lecture. Each branch can be extended with details illustrating or clarifying the subdivision. An example based on the theme of Chapter 4 of this book is shown in Figure 5.1.

Concept maps are a more difficult approach to note taking for students to learn but the graphical display makes it easier for students to learn the content when they use graphic organizers to study for tests. The best way to teach this skill is to model it. When working with individual students, it may be easier to teach concept mapping using a chapter from the student's text (e.g., social studies or science) before applying the method to lectures. Giving students partially completed concept maps and having them fill in the missing pieces is a way to shape the skill (or fade the support).

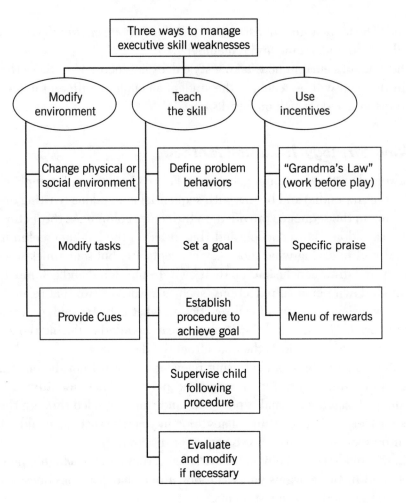

FIGURE 5.1. Example of a concept map.

Modifications for Whole-Class Use

Since the note-taking processes we've described require students to listen carefully to lectures and make decisions about what's important and what's not important and how the information should be organized to facilitate understanding and retention, we believe that this skill should be taught to all students. Suggestions for how to do this include:

1. In teaching the Cornell method, begin by providing a master copy of lecture notes with the center column completed. As the lecture progresses, stop periodically and ask students to pick out key terms and concepts and write them in the blank left-hand column on the master copy. Ask students to give examples of the kinds of personal reflections, questions, or examples of relationships to prior knowledge or personal experience and instruct them to write these down in the right-hand column.

2. For another class, provide a master copy that includes only the key terms and concepts but omits the running notes. Ask students to fill in that portion of the form as well as to add personal comments in the right-hand column. Walk around the room to spot check how students have done.

3. In teaching concept mapping, provide students with a concept map with only the main subdivisions filled in. As you lecture, turn your lecture into a concept map either on the blackboard or on an overhead projector. In subsequent classes, provide a blank concept map and ask students to fill it in as the lecture progresses. You may also want to ask students to complete concept maps on book chapters when assigning text reading for homework. In both cases, check work to see whether they understand how to organize concept maps.

4. Expose students to a variety of graphic organizers. Websites that provide downloadable examples are *www.edhelper.com*, *www.eduplace.com*, and *www.teachervision.fen.com*. Many others can be located by typing "graphic organizer" into a search engine such as Google.

5. After you have taught both note-taking strategies, ask students to select which one they prefer to use.

6. At the end of each class, ask students in groups of two or three to compare their notes to see whether they agree on the key concepts and to give them a chance to fill in any missing information.

7. For students with disabilities and those who can't keep up with note-taking demands, provide a master copy of the lecture notes and ask them to add to it their own personal comments. The Cornell method will probably work better for students with processing difficulties since it gives them a space to jot down key concepts and personal reflections.

13. LEARNING TO MANAGE EFFORTFUL TASKS

Executive Skills Addressed: *Task Initiation, Sustained Attention*

Most students are able to get through typical class assignments without much difficulty, because teachers adjust the assignment to match the attentional capacity and the skill level of the typical child at any given grade level. Some youngsters, however, find normal routine assignments exceedingly effortful and go to great lengths to avoid completing them. This routine is intended for this kind of student.

There are two primary ways to make tasks that the student sees as taking a lot of effort less aversive: Reduce the amount of effort required, by making it briefer or easier, or offer a large enough incentive that the child is willing to expend the effort required to get the reward. (See Chapter 4 for discussion of effortful tasks.) Examples of ways to do this are

1. Break down the task into very small parts, so that each part requires no more than X minutes. X is determined by the student's current performance. The rule of thumb is that, from the student's perspective, at the beginning of the task the end should be in sight. At the completion of the task, praise the student, and either give him or her a short break or a

chance to engage in a more preferred activity for a limited time. Alternatively, you can offer points or tokens that can later be redeemed for some preferred item or activity.

2. If possible, allow the student to decide how to break down the task. For example, give the student the choice of how many math problems he or she will complete before a break.

3. For more difficult tasks, give the student something more powerful to look forward to doing when the task is done. For instance, the student might earn 10 minutes of computer time for completing his or her class work in language arts within a specified time frame, and with an agreed-upon quality (such as making no more than two mistakes on grammar or spelling).

4. Reward the student for being willing to tackle tasks that demand effort. You could, for example, with the student draw up an academic task list (e.g., journal, math word problems) and have the student rate each task for effort required. In and of itself this is useful because it will help you identify those areas the student views as most difficult or effortful. It may be helpful to create a scale for effort—1 for the easiest tasks up to 10 for the hardest tasks the student could ever imagine doing. Once the student masters the use of the scale, you could work on thinking about how to turn a high-effort task (say, one rated 8–10) into a lower-effort task (one rated 3–4). Offering a more powerful incentive for undertaking more effortful tasks can help the student to better tolerate effort.

If approaches such as these don't help the student complete tough tasks without complaining, whining, crying, or otherwise resisting, you may want to take a slower and more labor-intensive approach to training the student to tolerate high-effort tasks. This approach, is called backward chaining.

Essentially, the student starts at the end of a high-effort task, at first completing only the very last step to earn a reward. This last step might be having the student write the last sentence of a paragraph before getting a break or receiving an incentive. This process would continue until the student can complete that step with minimal effort and then you would back up to do another step. Over time, the student is backed through the task until you get to the point where you expect him or her to complete the entire task independently. While school staff may be hesitant to use this approach because it is labor-intensive and slow in the early stages, for the reluctant and work-avoidant student, the backward chaining actually trains the student to tolerate tedious or high-effort work and eventually eliminates the need for constant cuing/nagging.

Modifications for Whole-Class Use

Discuss with the class as a group the notion of effortful tasks, and introduce them to the 10-point scale. Ask for opinions about what tasks they find easy or hard. Typically, this will lead to the discovery that what some students see as easy, others find hard. Have the same discussion about chores at home. Then solicit ideas about strategies they use to manage difficult tasks, and from these as well as your own ideas, create a classroom list of interventions that they can use when they come up against a difficult task. If students don't offer this themselves, ensure that asking for help from a peer or teacher is always an option. Have the students create their own personal lists of difficult tasks so that they can work on preempting avoidance, escape, or refusal of the task.

A somewhat light-hearted approach to encouraging students to tolerate effortful tasks might be to ask students to award themselves points based on how hard they had to work to make themselves get through the task, with more points allotted for effortful tasks and fewer points for those they can get through without difficulty. Make sure they understand the difference between *effortful* and *difficult*; otherwise, students may use the game as a way to boast about how easy they find schoolwork.

14. LEARNING TO CONTROL ONE'S TEMPER

Executive Skills Addressed: *Emotional Control, Response Inhibition, Flexibility*

We assume that if the behaviors are highly disruptive or involve physical aggression, then both a functional behavior assessment and a behavior support plan have been or will be completed. We have used the following intervention as a free standing plan for less serious behavior issues and as part of a behavior support plan for those that are more significant.

1. Together with the student, make a list of the things that happen that cause the student to lose his or her temper (these are called triggers). You may want to make a long list of all the different things that make the student angry and then see whether they can be grouped into larger categories (when told "No," when he or she is given difficult work, when something planned doesn't happen, etc.).

2. Talk with the student about what "losing your temper" looks or sounds like (e.g., yells, swears, throws things, hitting). Decide which ones of these should go on a "can't do" list. Keep this list short and work on only one or two behaviors at a time.

3. Now make a list of things the student can do instead (called replacement behaviors). These should be three or four different things the student can do instead of the "can't do" behaviors you've selected.

4. Put these on a "Hard Times Board." (Figure 5.2 is a completed sample, and form 5.11 is a blank version; see p. 210 in the Appendix.)

5. Practice. Say to the student, "Let's pretend you're upset because Billy wouldn't play with you at recess. Which strategy do you want to use?" (See the more detailed practice guidelines that follow.)

6. After practicing for a week or so with modeling and rehearsal, start using the process "for real," but initially use it for only minor irritants.

7. After using it successfully with minor irritants, move on to the more challenging triggers.

8. If the student is still struggling, connect the process to a reward. For best results, use two levels of rewards: a "bigger reward" for never getting to the point where the Hard Times Board needs to be used, and a "smaller reward" for successfully using a strategy on the Hard Time Board to deal with the trigger situation.

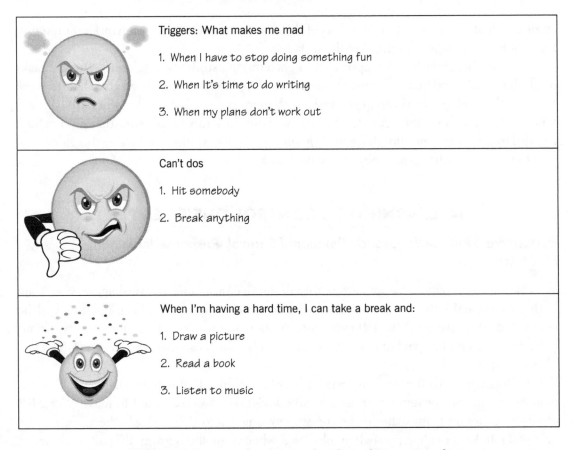

Triggers: What makes me mad

1. When I have to stop doing something fun

2. When It's time to do writing

3. When my plans don't work out

Can't dos

1. Hit somebody

2. Break anything

When I'm having a hard time, I can take a break and:

1. Draw a picture

2. Read a book

3. Listen to music

FIGURE 5.2. Example of a completed Hard Times Board.

Practicing the Procedure

1. Use real-life examples. These should include a variety representing the different categories of triggers.

2. Make the practice sessions "quick and dirty." For example, if a coping strategy is to read a book, have the student open a book and start reading, but don't spend more than 20–30 seconds on this.

3. Have the student practice each of the strategies listed on the Hard Times Board.

4. Have brief practice sessions daily or several times a week for a week or two before putting it into effect.

Modifications/Adjustments

1. At first you may need to model the use of the strategy. This means talking aloud to show what the child might be saying or thinking as he or she implements the strategy.

2. There may be times when, despite having a procedure in place, the student still loses control and can't calm down or use any of the strategies on the Hard Times Board. In this case, remove the student from the situation. Tell the student in advance that you will do

this so that the student knows what to expect. Say, "If you scream [hit, throw objects] we're always going to leave."

3. If the student is fairly consistently unable to use the strategies effectively, then a more involved behavior assessment and plan is needed.

Modifications for Whole-Class Use

Classroom and school rules typically will address behaviors associated with anger/temper outbursts. Whenever possible, we believe it is essential for executive skill development to involve children in the process of rule development and strategy generation to address these behaviors for the classroom and for the school. Obtaining peer input and a group consensus about rules and strategies gives children the opportunity to think in advance about such behaviors, creates student "buy-in," and helps students develop a sense of ownership and self-management. Having rules and strategies in place and regularly reviewing them with the class provides a proactive plan for managing such behaviors and makes it more likely that students will either inhibit these behaviors or utilize the agreed-upon strategies. We know teachers who post the strategies and refer children to them when the behaviors do occur. We also have observed classrooms and schools that have established peer-mediation/conflict mediation plans or programs to manage these behaviors when they are the result of interpersonal conflicts or situations that students deem unfair. Providing students of any age with an active, peer-managed, and institutionally acceptable method of resolving conflicts and complaints epitomizes the development of executive skills. Adults are available to act as models and to provide parameters for acceptable rules and strategies, students learn the decision-making process, and more responsibility can be given as executive skills and frontal lobes mature.

15. LEARNING TO CONTROL IMPULSIVE BEHAVIOR

Executive Skills Addressed: *Response Inhibition, Emotional Control*

1. Together with the student, identify the situations where the impulsive behavior occurs (circle, transitions between classes, gym, etc.).

2. Agree on a rule for the situations. The rule should focus on what the student can do to control impulses (raise hand, lower voice, keep hands to self). If possible, build in choice if you can; in other words, try to come up with a couple of different things he or she can do in place of the unwanted impulsive response. (See Form 5.12 on p. 211 of the Appendix.)

3. Cue the student to repeat the expectation and decide about what you might do to signal the student that you think he or she is on the verge of "losing control" so that he or she can back off or use one of the agreed-upon behaviors or strategies. This works best when the signal is a relatively discrete visual signal (e.g., a hand motion) that can alert the student to the potential problem situation.

4. Practice the procedure. Make this a "Let's pretend" role play: "Let's pretend we're at circle doing sharing time and you have something you really want to share but there are

six other children before you. Tell me/show me what you can do to help you wait for your turn."

5. As with the other skills involving behavior regulation, practice the procedure daily or several times a week for a couple of weeks.

6. When you and the student are ready to put the procedure in effect in "real life," remind him or her about it just before the trigger situation is likely to occur (e.g., "Remember the plan," "Tell me what you're going to do.").

7. Review how the process worked afterward. You may want to create a scale that you and the student can use to assess how well it went (5—Went without a hitch! to 1—That didn't go real well!).

Modifications/Adjustments

1. If you think it will make the process work more effectively or more quickly, tie the successful use of a replacement behavior to a reinforcer. This may best be done using a "response cost" approach. For example, give the student 70 points to begin the day. Each time the student acts impulsively, subtract 10 points. You can also give bonus points if the student gets through a specified period of time without losing any points.

2. If impulsivity is a significant problem for the student, begin by choosing one time of day or one impulsive behavior to target to make success more likely.

3. Be sure to praise the student for showing self-control. Even if you're using tangible rewards, social praise should always accompany any other kind of reinforcer.

Modifications for Whole-Class Use

As is the case with anger control above, many of the behaviors associated with self-control will be dealt with through classroom rules. For example, talking out, interrupting, and talking over other people is a common complaint from teachers. Students want to be heard first. Giving students the opportunity to experience firsthand the problems that this causes can help set the stage of discussion of classroom rules. To demonstrate this, we know one teacher who assigns passages for children to read aloud and when they each have a passage, she tells them to begin reading. After 1 minute she has them stop and asks the group questions about the different passages. They quickly discover that they are not able to answer most of the questions, leading to a discussion of why and what would help solve the problem.

Maintaining personal space in close quarters (morning meeting, waiting in line, cafeteria) creates another situation that often leads to impulsive behavior (touching, pushing, poking, etc.) for some children. Working on the idea of personal space initially happens by talking with children concretely about what it means (e.g., arm's length away when face to face, no physical contact in circle) and having them suggest ways to find a solution. Since space is the issue, having some physical reminder (carpet squares, placement of desks, number of seats at a table, maintain a set distance in line) is often helpful. We also have worked with teachers who, in the context of this discussion, help the class agree on a few signals (usually gestures since they are less obtrusive) to let peers know when they need space. This is especially important as children get older since the "rules" for personal space are tied more to relationships among peers. What might be entirely acceptable for physical contact between some peers does not extend to any member of the group. Hence, modeling what one's peers are doing can lead to significant problems if a student doesn't understand the social context. As with the other interventions we have discussed, it is important to review rules and expectations regularly, especially before students enter situations where the level of stimulation and/or physical proximity makes impulsive behavior more likely.

16. LEARNING TO MANAGE ANXIETY

Executive Skills Addressed: Emotional Control, Flexibility

1. Together with the student, make a list of the things that happen that cause him or her to feel anxious. In school, certain situations/tasks account for many of the worries that students experience. These include the following:

- Going into or anticipating a new situation (e.g., school, classroom, teacher, peers)
- Going into large, less structured, high-stimulation situations where there is less adult supervision (e.g., cafeteria)
- Being called on in class, particularly in a weak subject area
- Being teased or bullied
- Giving an oral report
- Taking a test
- Finding one's way around (particularly in middle or high school)
- Asking a question when unsure about the subject/problem and so on
- Changes in schedule

Identifying the specific source of worry is a key first step in helping the student to develop a plan to manage the anxiety.

2. Talk with the student about what anxiety feels like so he or she can recognize it in the early stages. This is often a physical feeling—"butterflies" in the stomach, sweaty hands, faster heartbeat.

3. Now make a list of things the student can do instead of thinking about the worry. This is a two-step process. After working with the student to identify the source, the teacher or school counselor and the student will discuss a strategy that might involve gradual exposure to a situation (e.g., a series of visits to a new class) or development of a study plan (e.g., for test anxiety). In some cases, such as teasing/bullying, a good part of the problem resolution rests primarily with an adult. Having addressed the trigger, the next step involves helping the student develop techniques that are calming or divert attention from the worries since it is unlikely that addressing the trigger alone will alleviate the feelings. The "Modifications/ Adjustments" paragraph below describes some of these.

4. Put these strategies on a "Worry Board." (Figure 5.3 is a completed sample, and Form 5.13 is a blank version; see p. 212 in the Appendix.)

5. Practice. How practice is done depends on the problem. For recurring but infrequent triggers such as moving to a new class, the same or similar strategies can be used from year to year if they have been effective. We work with some students whose transition

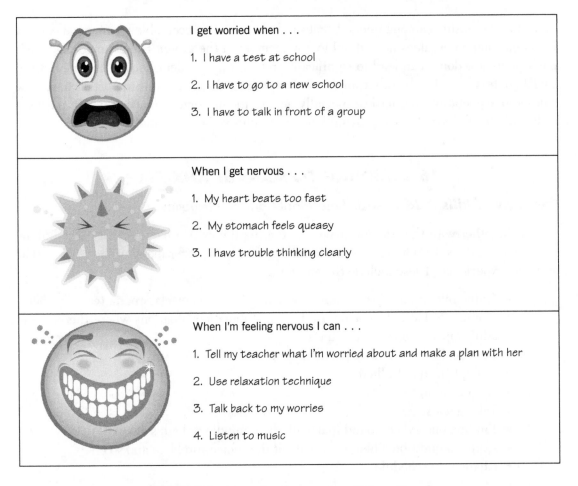

I get worried when . . .

1. I have a test at school

2. I have to go to a new school

3. I have to talk in front of a group

When I get nervous . . .

1. My heart beats too fast

2. My stomach feels queasy

3. I have trouble thinking clearly

When I'm feeling nervous I can . . .

1. Tell my teacher what I'm worried about and make a plan with her

2. Use relaxation technique

3. Talk back to my worries

4. Listen to music

FIGURE 5.3. Example of a completed Worry Board.

plan every year involves early and repeated visits to the receiving classroom. In other cases, for example going into the cafeteria, practice may involve gradual exposure (going in for a short time or initially when there are only a few students present). The general approach involves what is called guided mastery in which the degree of anxiety to which the student is exposed is low enough so that with some support he or she can get through it successfully. The exposure has to be very gradual; you don't move to the next step until the student feels comfortable with the current step. The critical elements in guided mastery are physical distance and time. At the outset, the student is far removed from the anxiety-provoking object or situation and the exposure is for a very short time. The distance is then reduced and the time increases gradually.

It's also helpful to have a script (something the student is to say in the situation) and a tactic he or she can use (such as relaxation, thought stopping or something he or she can do to divert his or her attention—see below for a description of these). Regular practice with these techniques is needed if they are to be reliable for the student. Initially they need to be practiced in the absence of significant anxiety or worry. As the student becomes more practiced and proficient in their use, they can be used in situations of greater anxiety. However, the process must, like guided mastery, be very gradual. The usefulness of the technique for the student is judged by his or her ability to successfully reduce the worry or anxiety felt in a situation to a lower level.

Modifications/Adjustments

Possible coping strategies for managing anxiety might include deep or slow breathing, counting to 20, or using other relaxation strategies; thought stopping or talking back to your worries, drawing a picture of the worry, folding it up, and putting it in a box with a lid; listening to music (and maybe dancing to it); or challenging the logic of the worry. For further explanation of these strategies, google "Relaxation for Kids" and check out the websites that come up. Another helpful resource is a book written for students and parents to read together: *What to Do When You Worry Too Much* by Dawn Huebner, PhD (2006).

17. MANAGING CHANGES IN PLANS OR SCHEDULES

Executive Skills Addressed: *Emotional Control, Flexibility*

Helping a child accept changes in plans without anger or distress involves some advance work and lots of practice. Whenever possible, the student needs to know the schedule or agenda ahead of time, before he or she has formulated a plan for that time period. Meanwhile, you start introducing the student to small changes on a regular basis, gradually increasing the student's tolerance for changes over time.

1. Schools and classrooms typically have well-rehearsed schedules and routines. Nonetheless, for students who are anxious about change, we have seen problems develop when teachers want to be flexible and take advantage of "teachable moments," at the various times of the year when routines do change (e.g., holiday activities, assemblies, special visitors) and when there are substitute teachers. Letting students know in advance that these changes will happen during the year and providing, when possible, some advance preparation such as the day before or the day of the activity, or even a few minutes before the actual change will help.

2. Try not to attach precise times to the activities unless necessary (as with sports events and lessons), using time ranges instead. For example, the popcorn party the class has earned as a reward will take place "sometime after lunch."

3. Talk with the student about the fact that changes or "surprises" can always come up despite plans and schedules established in advance. Give examples (indoor recess on a rainy day, a teacher being absent, fire alarms)

4. Create a visual for the schedule, such as activities written on a card or a series of pictures, and post it in the room. Make a "Surprise!" card (see Form 5.14A on p. 213 in the Appendix) for the schedule and explain that when a change is coming, you will show him or her the card, say what the change is, and put it on the schedule. (Even when a change comes up that's a surprise to everyone, you can pull out the card and follow the same process.)

5. Review the schedule with the class at the beginning of the day.

6. Start to introduce changes and show the Surprise! card. Initially, these should be pleasant, such as extra snack or recess time, free time during class to do homework, and so on. Gradually introduce more "neutral" changes (math before reading) Eventually, include less pleasant changes (can't do a planned activity because of weather, pop quizzes).

If the Surprise! card and the gradual introduction of changes are not sufficient, there are a few other approaches to consider. When possible, introduce the change well before the event. This gives the student time to adjust gradually rather than quickly. Depending on his or her reaction to less pleasant change (crying, resisting, complaining), talk about other behaviors the student could use that would allow for protest in an acceptable way, such as filling out a "Complaint Form" (see Form 5.14B on p. 213 in the Appendix). You also can provide a reward for successfully managing the change. Keep in mind that reactivity to change decreases with the amount of exposure that the student has and the success he or she has in negotiating it. As long as the exposure is gradual and does not initially involve situations that are frustrating or threatening, the student can become more flexible.

18. LEARNING NOT TO CRY OVER LITTLE THINGS

Executive Skills Addressed: *Emotional Control, Flexibility*

This is generally not an issue past lower elementary school, but when students cry over little things, they may be trying to get attention or help, trying to avoid a task/situation or a change or to express a feeling (frustration, fear, anger, etc). So the goal of this intervention is not to teach kids to be tough little soldiers or anything of the sort, but to help them find ways other than crying to get what they want/need. The goal is to get them to use words instead of tears in those situations where crying does not appear to be an appropriate response.

1. Establish, through a functional analysis, what the motivation is for the behavior and the tasks/situations that are most likely to trigger it.

2. Explain that the student needs to use words instead of tears when upset. This can be done by having the child use a functional communication to indicate the need or feeling ("I need help," "I don't want to do this," "I'm upset," "I'm sad," "I'm angry," etc.).

3. If it's a feelings issue caused by frustration, let the student know that it may be helpful for him or her to say what caused these feelings (for example, "I'm upset because I wanted to play four-square but he was playing tag" or "I'm mad because I lost the game").

4. When the student is able to use words, respond by validating his or her feelings (for example, "I can see you're upset. Not being able to play with a friend must be a big disappointment to you"). Statements like this will communicate to the student that you understand and sympathize.

5. Let the student know in advance what will happen when an upsetting situation arrives. This should include giving him or her a script for handling the situation. You might say, "When you feel like crying, you can use words like 'I'm angry,' 'I'm sad,' 'I need help,' or 'I need a break.' When you use words, I'll listen and try to help or understand your feelings. If you start to cry, though, I can't help because I don't know what you need. When

you can use your words, we can talk." At first you may periodically need to remind the student of the procedure to prepare him or her to follow the script when an upsetting situation occurs.

6. If the student starts to cry, make sure he or she gets no attention from anyone for crying. This means no attention from anyone (staff, peers, etc.), so you should make sure everyone likely to be involved understands the procedure. Without the attention for crying, it will gradually diminish (although it may get worse initially before it gets better).

7. The goal here is obviously not to extinguish all crying (because there are legitimate reasons for students to cry). A rule of thumb for judging when it may be appropriate to cry is to think about the average peer of the student's age. Would crying be a natural response in the situation at hand?

Modifications/Adjustments

If crying is firmly entrenched, you may want to build in a reinforcer to help the child learn to use words instead of tears. Depending on the age of the student, you could give him or her stickers or points for using words instead of tears or for going a certain amount of time without crying. To determine how long that time should be, it would be helpful to take a baseline so you know how frequently the student cries now. An "Upset Log" to help you track how often the crying occurs, how long it lasts, and what the precipitating event is included to help you do this. Following the log is a "Contract" you can make with the student to handle crying. Depending on the age of the student, the contract can be completed with words, pictures, or both. (See Forms 5.15A and B on p. 214 in the Appendix.)

19. LEARNING TO SOLVE PROBLEMS

Executive Skills Addressed: Metacognition, Flexibility, Planning

1. Talk with the student about what the problem is. This generally involves three steps:

- Empathizing with the student or letting him or her know you understand how he or she feels ("I can see that makes you really mad" or "That must be really upsetting for you")
- Getting a *general* sense of what the problem is ("Let me get this straight—you're upset because the friend you were hoping to play with at recess doesn't want to play with you")
- Defining the problem more narrowly so that you can begin to brainstorm solutions ("You're not sure what to do when you go out to recess").

2. Brainstorm solutions. Together with the student, think of as many different things as you can that might solve the problem. You may want to set a time limit (like 2 minutes) since this sometimes speeds up the process or makes it feel less like an open-ended task. Write down all the possible solutions. Don't criticize the solutions at this point, since this tends to squelch the creative thinking process.

3. Ask the student to look at all the solutions and pick the one he or she likes best. You may want to start by having him or her circle the top three to five choices and then narrow them down by talking about the pluses and minuses associated with each choice.

4. Ask the student if he or she needs help carrying out the choice.

5. Talk about what will happen if the first solution doesn't work. This may involve choosing a different solution or analyzing where the first solution went wrong and fixing it.

6. Praise him or her for coming up with a good solution (and then praise again after the solution is implemented).

This is a standard problem-solving approach that can be used for all kinds of problems, including interpersonal problems as well as obstacles that prevent a student from getting what he or she wants or needs. Sometimes the best solution will involve figuring out ways to overcome the obstacles, while at other times it may involve helping the student come to terms with the fact that he or she cannot have what he or she wants.

Sometimes the problem-solving process may lead to a "negotiation," in which you and the student both agree on what will be done to reach a solution that's mutually satisfactory. In this case, you should explain to the student that whatever solution you come up with, you both have to be able to live with it. You may want to talk about how labor contracts are negotiated so that both workers and bosses get something they want out of the bargain.

After you've used the process (and the worksheet) with the student for a number of different kinds of problems, the student may be able to use the worksheet independently. Since your goal should be to foster independent problem solving, you may want to ask the student to fill out the Solving Problems Worksheet alone before coming to you for your help (if needed). Eventually, the student will internalize the whole process and be able to solve problems "on the fly." (See Form 5.16 on p. 215 in the Appendix for a blank worksheet.)

Modifications for Whole-Class Use

This is an ideal methodology to teach whole classrooms. Everyone can benefit from learning a procedure for solving problems. The one described here, once the class has learned the steps, can be used by teachers whenever a problem comes up. Furthermore, it can be applied to both academic and social problems. Students can be asked to use the process individually or they can be assigned a buddy to help them. Problem solving is also an excellent small-group exercise. In this case, group members can be assigned different roles to play: one student may be asked to lead the discussion, another to take notes, and a third to make sure the rules are enforced. Teachers are also encouraged to ask students to evaluate how the process has worked so that students learn to evaluate the quality of the solutions they have come up with.

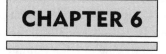

CHAPTER 6

Interventions for Specific Executive Skills Domains

Now we turn to interventions designed to enhance specific executive skills. These interventions have been "field tested," and we are satisfied, based on parent and teacher feedback, that they fit well with real-world demands. Nonetheless, keep in mind that the suggestions provided will not work with all children and that adaptations will need to be made particularly with respect to the developmental level of the child or the severity of the problem.

As a general metaphor to help readers understand the process of enhancing executive skills, think of these tools as ways to assist children on a journey. The kinds of modifications and strategies we describe below can be thought of as ways to shorten the journey, help travelers see their destination more clearly, give them signposts to let them know they're on the right road and to mark their progress, give them a "roadmap" to guide them, or maybe even a global positioning system spelling out more precisely where they are and where they need to go next.

Think for a moment about the concept of a roadmap. A roadmap provides directions for how to get from a starting point to an ending point. If I don't know how to get some place, I have someone draw me a map. In the beginning, I need to bring that map with me and refer to it frequently so I don't get lost. But if I go to that same place often enough, I no longer need the map. This is because I've *internalized* the map and can rely on my own mental representation of the directions to get me where I need to go. This same approach applies to improving executive skills. Initially, we draw a map for children and we prompt them to refer to the map so they don't get lost. With practice, they no longer need either the map or the external cues because they have internalized them and can follow the procedure on their own.

The remainder of this chapter presents one table for each executive skill (Tables 6.1–6.11). Each table includes the following components: (1) suggested environmental modifications that can be put in place for the youngster with a weakness in that executive skill area,

(2) examples of steps or procedures that can be followed to teach the skill, and (3) a brief vignette that illustrates an application of environmental modifications or skill instruction to a typical home or school situation in which the executive skill might be displayed. We follow each vignette with a brief list of "Keys to Success," which provide additional pointers to be kept in mind when implementing an intervention like the one described in the vignette.

We need to caution readers not to look at what follows as a "cookbook" designed to produce solutions to very specific problems. Rather, we hope that readers recognize that executive skill deficits will incur problems that arise *across* situations. For instance, youngsters with time management problems generally don't just have problems managing their time in order to complete schoolwork; they generally also have difficulty managing their time in other arenas—completing chores, getting to appointments on time, deciding how they are going to spend their free time, and so on. As you read through the following section, we encourage you to consider executive skill weakness more broadly and how it comes into play in specific situations in a youngster's daily life.

We also should note that while each executive skill has unique aspects to it, there are common interventions that apply across executive skills in some cases. For this reason, some interventions will be mentioned in more than one table or the reader will be referred to related skills for additional suggestions.

TABLE 6.1. Response Inhibition

Description of skill

The capacity to think before you act; the capacity to delay or inhibit responding based on the ability to evaluate multiple factors. Children who have trouble with response inhibition are impulsive, saying or doing things without thinking, which often gets them into trouble with parents, teachers, or peers.

Environmental modifications

- Increase external controls, in other words, restrict access to settings or situations in which the child can get in trouble. A child who becomes overstimulated during physical education classes and has trouble following class rules may need close supervision during these classes. Children who have trouble keeping their hands to themselves or their bodies stationary during circle time benefit from sitting next to the teacher or an adult who can use nonverbal cues (e.g., a hand on the arm) to keep them settled.
- Increase supervision. When parents say, "I can't let him out of my sight," this suggests they have modified the environment by making sure there is an adult present at all times to reduce the likelihood that the child will do something dangerous or forbidden. Children with impulse control problems, particularly when they are young, often require more adult supervision in school settings. This is why the adult-to-student ratio is greater in preschools than in middle school. It is also why schools will sometimes assign individual aides to children. The physical presence of an adult in proximity to the child with impulse control problems acts as a cue for the child to exercise control.
- Find ways to cue the child to control impulses. This may include posting and reviewing class rules or stopping a child before he or she goes out to recess to ask, "What behavior are we working on?" to remind the child to exhibit self-control in specific situations (the child might say in answer to that question, "Not hitting when I get mad").

Teaching the skill

Focus of instruction: to teach the child a competing skill to replace the disinhibited response. For instance, if blurting out in class is the problem, then teach the child to raise his or her hand before speaking.

Steps to follow:
1. Explain to the child the skill being worked on and your understanding of the intent of the child's behavior (e.g., "I think you talk out because you're looking for recognition from me or your classmates. We're going to work on raising your hand before you speak"). In selecting the replacement skill (e.g., hand raising), make sure the skill being taught meets the same need (i.e., peer or teacher recognition).
2. Walk the child through the process, having him or her practice the skills using a contrived situation or a teaching example. Practice the skill sufficiently so that the child can be successful most of the time (you may want to make a game of the process, such as a variation of "Simon Says"). For instance, if hand raising is the skill being taught, then the practice could include keeping score for how many times the child remembers to raise his or her hand before speaking during the practice sessions.
3. At the point when the child is ready to use the skill in the natural environment, the child should be cued to use the skill just prior to the situation in which the skill will be required (e.g., by saying to the child, "Remember what we're working on").
4. Reinforce the child immediately for using the skill (e.g., if hand raising is the skill being taught, then early in the training stage, call on the child right away whenever the child raises his or her hand and praise the child for remembering to do so).

(cont.)

109

TABLE 6.1. *(cont.)*

5. Ignore the disinhibited response (e.g., don't respond when he or she blurts out).
6. Gradually fade the cuing and reinforcement (e.g., by not calling on the child right away every time she raises his or her hand is raised). This may be even more effective if you tell the child that this is what you are going to do (e.g., "I'm not going to call on you every time. I won't forget you're there, but I'm only going to call on you every fourth or fifth time.").

Vignette

Circle time was a constant struggle for 7-year-old Kristin and her teacher, Ms. Brock. In spite of rules about turn taking and not interrupting every day, Kristin would blurt out information when someone else was talking instead of raising her hand and waiting to be called on. Ms. Brock decided that providing some cues and a plan for Kristin could help. She first introduced a "talking stick" to the class and indicated that only the person who had the stick could speak at that moment. She also gave two chips to each child that he or she could "spend" by asking two questions once the speaker indicated it was time for questions. At this point, the children would raise their hands and the teacher would call on one. Recognizing that Kristin had difficulty waiting, for the first week the teacher called on her first. If Kristin forgot and blurted something out before the speaker was finished, she had to give up one of her chips. This, along with initially sitting next to the teacher, was usually sufficient to help her remember. However, on a few occasions Kristin (and a few other children) "spent" both chips before the speaker was done and needed to leave the circle. Kristin found this system helpful, and after the first week she was able to decide with her teacher how many children she felt she could wait for before asking her questions.

Keys to success

1. Have the student practice the skill in a classroom situation (either academic or social, as appropriate to the skill being taught).
2. If using a chip system, let the child participate in the decision about how many chips he or she needs.
3. Review the rules and expectations just before entering the situation where the behavior typically occurs (e.g., "Tell me what you're working on").
4. Have the child rate his or her performance to build self-evaluation skills.

TABLE 6.2. Working Memory

Description of skill

The ability to hold information in mind while performing complex tasks. It incorporates the ability to draw on past learning or experience to apply to the situation at hand or to project into the future.

Environmental modifications

These are usually either storage mechanisms or cuing mechanisms, designed to help the child store information in memory (or in some other more readily retrievable location, such as a calendar or notebook) or to cue the child to retrieve the information on demand or at a set time.

Storage devices include the following:
- Agenda books or calendars (e.g., for writing down assignments or appointments).
- Notebooks (e.g., for keeping to-do lists).
- Electronic devices such as Palm Pilots, tape recorders, or message systems (e.g., some people call their answering machines to remind them of things they need to do when they get home; others use electronic messaging devices). Smart phones such as iPhones have both built-in storage capacities (such as a note function) as well as additional applications such as homework-tracking programs that can be downloaded for free or for a small price at the iTunes Store.

Cuing devices include the following:
- Arranging for verbal reminders (e.g., from parent, teacher, aide, or peer).
- Page systems.
- Alarms on watches (some watches allow for multiple alarms) or on cell phones.
- Visual cues displayed in a prominent place (writing on the back of one's hand, Post-it software for the computer desktop, etc.).
- Taking advantage of a naturally occurring cue in the environment. This can be manipulated by placing the cue in a prominent place where it's not likely to be missed. For example, if a child has trouble remembering to take morning medication, he or she could place the pill bottle directly in front of the box of cereal on the breakfast table. Another example would be to incorporate recurring phrases teachers might use or teacher behaviors (e.g., using the music teacher's tapping his baton on the desk to bring the class to order as a signal to a child to stop talking).

For cues to be effective, they should ideally be unusual or unexpected so that they do not blend into their surroundings. Auditory cues tend to be more effective than visual ones, because they're more likely to cause the individual to attend to the cue (if only to ask, "What's *that*?"). It's also possible to increase the salience of the cue by having the child practice responding to it.

Teaching the skill

Rather than assigning cues, teach the child to design his or her own cues and to put systems in place to use the cues. The steps to follow are
1. Explain the problem as it shows in the child.
2. With younger children, give them a range of options and have them pick one that's appealing. Or have them generate their own.
3. Mentally rehearse the association between the cue and the working memory. Then use *in vivo* rehearsal.
4. Devise a monitoring system (e.g., "Did you use the cue?" [Yes/No.] "How well did you do?").

(cont.)

111

TABLE 6.2. *(cont.)*

Vignette

Mario, age 11, was continually forgetting things he needed to bring home from school, such as his homework, assignment book, and permission slips to be signed. His mother kept having to drive him back to school to collect the things he forgot. She did this for a while; then she felt she was rewarding him for forgetting, so she stopped. Sometimes he would earn a lower grade on his homework or he would have to serve a detention for forgetting assignments, but this didn't seem to help him remember. His mother met with his teacher to see if there might be a better way to handle the problem. Together, Mario's mother and teacher and Mario himself developed a list of the things he might need to remember to bring home each day. His teacher added some things he tended to forget to do during the school day as well (see Form 5.2 the End of Day Checklist on p 199 in the Appendix). They placed the checklist in a plastic sleeve and had Mario use a pen that could be erased after he completed the checklist each day. During the last 10 minutes of the school day, a teacher aide and Mario went through the checklist item by item. For quite a while, the aide needed to stay with Mario to make sure he completed the entire checklist. Eventually, she was able just to prompt Mario to "get out your checklist" and to check with him after he'd completed it.

Keys to success

1. Be thorough and positive with the child, particularly in the early stages of teaching the skill.
2. Err on the side of cuing for too long. If discontinued too soon, the child will not have time to internalize the process.
3. Ensure the child has set aside time to actually do the monitoring.

TABLE 6.3. Emotional Control

Description of skill

The ability to manage emotions in order to achieve goals, complete tasks, or control and direct behavior.

Environmental modifications

These are designed to help students manage their emotions (both positive and negative) more effectively. They include the following:

- Anticipating problem situations and preparing child for them.
- Teaching coping strategies. For example, children who get anxious before exams can learn relaxation techniques.
- Giving children scripts to follow in target situations or things they can say to themselves to help them manage emotions.
- Structuring the environment to avoid problem situations or to intervene early. For example, if children become overstimulated in social situations, then limit the number of children they play with or increase the structure of the play activity.
- Breaking tasks into smaller steps to make them more manageable.
- Giving the child a break if a task appears to be becoming upsetting.
- Having adults model the practice of making positive self-statements. For instance, a parent or teacher might say to the child, "Here's what I want you to say to yourself before starting this: 'I know this will be hard for me, but I'm going to keep trying. If I get stuck after trying hard, I will ask for help.'"
- Giving "pep talks" to the child before beginning a task.
- Teaching the child that how you think about an experience can affect how you feel about that experience. Examples from sports psychology for older children or superheroes for younger children may be a good way to do this.
- Using literature (such as *The Little Engine That Could*) or writing individualized social stories to teach emotional control.
- Using 5-point scales to help students both identify their feelings and give them coping strategies for managing them so they don't get out of control. This involves rating the behavior of concern on a scale from 1 to 5, with either extreme representing the most positive or the most negative manifestation of the behavior. Each number between the two extremes is then labeled as representing an intermediate level of severity. Children can be taught to rate their own behavior and can be guided to reduce the severity of the feeling or behavior. Alternatively, each number on the scale can be associated with a different intervention. For an excellent guide to using 5-point scales with children with emotional problems, see *The Incredible 5-Point Scale* (Buron & Curtis, 2003).

Teaching the skill

This involves teaching the child to independently use strategies such as those described above. For example, the child could be taught to identify and use a coping strategy when he or she encounters a problem situation or the child could be taught to use other strategies such as breaking down a task, creating a script, or making positive self-statements. A general outline for teaching this kind of skill is

1. Explain the skill to the child.
2. Have the child practice the skill.
3. Reinforce the child for practicing well.
4. Cue the child to use the skill in real-life situations (classroom or home settings).
5. Reinforce the child for using the skill successfully.

(cont.)

TABLE 6.3. *(cont.)*

Specific strategies that children can be taught to use include:

- Self-statements to promote a positive emotional response or an effective coping strategy.
- Having the child verbalize a goal behavior ("Today I will _____") before entering the situation where he or she can display the goal behavior.
- The use of visual imagery. Here, teach the child to visualize him- or herself managing the problem situation successfully. For example, if the child tends to be a poor sport on the athletic field, have the child picture the umpire calling him or her out on a questionable strike and then have the child picture him- or herself walking back to the dugout with a calm facial expression.
- Having the child incorporate practicing the skill into something he or she does routinely every day (e.g., journal writing at school or a bedtime routine where the child describes a positive use of the skill to a parent who puts him or her to bed at night).

Vignette

Recess was often a traumatic time for Timmy, age 6. He loved swinging on a particular swing, but it was often in use by someone else when he got out to the playground. Once he got the swing for himself, he resisted giving it up to let someone else swing. The teacher on duty finally decided the best way to handle it was to teach Timmy a strategy for managing his emotions. She made a deal with Timmy that he could use the swing for the first 5 minutes of recess and then, if he gave up the swing to another child without a fight, he could swing again for the last 3 minutes of recess. She taught Timmy to say to himself, "If I don't get mad, I can have another turn" as he got off the swing. Before they used this plan at recess, she took Timmy out to the playground on his own to practice getting off the swing and saying the statement about not getting mad. They practiced this several times until Timmy thought he would be able to do it successfully at recess. Both during the practice sessions and once they started following the procedure at recess, his teacher praised him for following the plan successfully. In time, she taught Timmy to wait for a turn at the beginning of recess by saying to himself, "I can wait; it will be my turn soon." Before the year was over, Timmy was even able to invite other children to use his favorite swing and to give up his own turn to let someone else swing.

Keys to success

1. When teaching children to manage emotions, use the actual situations likely to trigger the emotional response (e.g., recess, contact with a specific child).
2. Work with the child to help him or her brainstorm a plan to manage the situation.
3. In the early stages of the plan, an adult should cue and provide support when the child enters the situation.
4. Adult and child should jointly evaluate the outcome and discuss changes in plans.

TABLE 6.4. Sustained Attention

Description of skill

The capacity to maintain attention to a situation or task in spite of distractibility, fatigue, or boredom.

Environmental modifications

These are designed either to accommodate to students' difficulty with sustained attention or to make it easier for them to attend longer to tasks. They might include the following:

- Writing start and stop times on assigned tasks to help students persist with tasks long enough to complete them.
- Using incentive systems. For youngsters who have no interest in the work they're being asked to do, extrinsic rewards are sometimes the best hope for success. To be effective, they need to be powerful, frequent, and varied. Examples include awarding points for completed work or for work completed within specific time parameters, or arranging for a preferred activity to immediately follow less attractive tasks in order to give the student something to look forward to.
- Breaking tasks into subtasks and giving the student short breaks after each subtask.
- Setting a kitchen timer and challenging the student to complete the task within the time allotted.
- Using a self-monitoring tape (an audiotape that sounds electronic tones at random intervals) and asking the student to ask him- or herself, "Was I paying attention?" each time the tone sounds.
- Choosing the time of day carefully (e.g., having children do difficult tasks at the time of day when they are most alert).
- Providing supervision. Youngsters attend best in situations in which they receive one-to-one attention, frequent feedback, and immediate reinforcement. Research also suggests that children with problems with sustained attention have less difficulty when working with fathers than when working with mothers. This may have implications for who supervises homework.
- Making tasks interesting for students, since people work longer and harder on tasks of interest to them than on those they consider tedious, boring, or not important. Ways to do this may include making the task active or interactive, or turning the task into a challenge, a game, or a contest.
- Giving the child something to look forward to that can be done as soon as the task is finished (e.g., allowing a seventh grader the chance to "instant message" his or her friends as soon as homework is done).
- Providing attention and praise when the student is on task.

Teaching the skill

Teaching children to sustain attention involves teaching them to internalize the externally imposed strategies described above. This can be done by

1. Helping youngsters become aware of their own attentional capacity (e.g., how long they can work before they need a break).
2. Teaching them how to break down a task into pieces that fit their attentional capacity.
3. Helping them make a work plan. This should include helping them allocate work according to their capacity, but it should also include helping them identify both motivational strategies and environmental cues they can use to help them stay on task. Motivational strategies might include finding ways to make the task more active (e.g., not just *reading* a social studies chapter but posing a question to read for, note taking, creating a graphic organizer, or highlighting) or creating a script to keep them going (the son of one of the authors used to tell himself, "You *can't* walk away from this" when he found his attention flagging during homework). Environmental cues might include setting kitchen timers or alarm clocks, or asking an adult to check in on them periodically to make sure they're working.
4. Cuing them to follow the plan they've devised.
5. Reinforcing them for following the plan successfully.
6. Gradually transferring the responsibility for making the plan to the students themselves.

(cont.)

115

TABLE 6.4. *(cont.)*

Vignette

Sarah, a fourth grader, had the hardest time getting her seatwork done. When the teacher assigned a task, she might start it right away, but she would become quickly distracted. She might get up and sharpen her pencil, go to the bathroom, or talk to the other students sitting at her table. Sometimes she might overhear a conversation at the next table and feel like she had to participate in that discussion. Her teacher used to keep her in from recess to finish her work or to send it home for homework, but her parents raised objections to this. So she decided to try a different approach. She sat down with Sarah and explained that getting her work done on time was important. She asked Sarah to think about what makes it hard to get her work done. Sarah was able to generate a long list; she included things like "My pencil lead breaks; other kids' talking distracts me; I get tired; sometimes I don't know how to do the work; I get bored; my hand gets tired of writing." The more they talked, the more it became apparent that the main reasons Sarah wasn't getting work done were because she got distracted and she thought the work was tedious. Her teacher decided it would be good to involve her parents in this, in part because they were resistant to her missing recess and bringing unfinished work home at night. All together they came up with two interventions: (1) Sarah's parents agreed that any day she came home with all her work done, she could watch a favorite daily TV show that she was usually only able to watch on school vacations; and (2) Sarah agreed to work on trying to pay attention better. Her teacher brought out the self-monitoring tape and explained how it worked. She combined the tape with a checklist so that whenever the tone sounded, Sarah was to circle "Yes" or "No" on the checklist to indicate whether she was paying attention. This was quite successful. After a period of time, the teacher removed the checklist and had Sarah just ask herself whether she was paying attention each time she heard the tone. The third step in fading the intervention was to place a sticker on Sarah's desk to use both as a cue to pay attention and as a reminder to ask herself if she was paying attention. Gradually Sarah was able to improve her efficient work production because of better attention.

Keys to success

1. If work completion remains an issue after instituting this kind of intervention, consider further modifying the task.
2. Use the Premack Principle (the less preferred task precedes the more preferred task).
3. Ensure that the child can "see" past the task to the preferred activity. Ask the child, "What do you get to do as soon as you finish this?"
4. If the child does not succeed quickly with this kind of intervention, add an incentive system.

TABLE 6.5. Task Initiation

<u>Description of skill</u>

The ability to begin a task without undue procrastination, in a timely fashion.

<u>Environmental modifications</u>

These are designed to help children get right to work when tasks are assigned or to begin them at a predetermined time. They include the following:

- Verbally cuing the child to get started.
- Arranging for a visual cue to prompt the child to begin (e.g., a picture taped to the desk).
- Walking the child through the first portion of the task to get him or her started.
- Noting start and stop times when tasks are assigned/completed.
- Having the child specify when he or she will begin the task and then cuing the child when the scheduled time arrives (this approach can be used quite successfully for homework or chores). Alternatively, have the child decide how he or she will be cued to begin the task (e.g., by using an alarm clock or a naturally occurring event to act as the cue, such as "immediately after lunch").

<u>Teaching the skill</u>

There are two kinds of task initiation: The first involves beginning a task right away when it is assigned and the second involves planning when a task will be done and starting it promptly at the predetermined time.

To begin tasks promptly, teach the child either to self-instruct (i.e., talk to him- or herself by saying something like "The teacher told us what to do and now it's time to start") or to perform right away the first step in the assigned task (open the textbook, get out pencil and paper, write his or her name at the top of the paper, etc.).

Teaching a child to begin a task promptly at some future predetermined time can be done with the following steps:

1. Have the child make a written plan for doing the task. This may include writing down the assignment and deciding on a start time. For longer projects, it may mean breaking the task down into subtasks and assigning start times to each subtask.
2. Have the child determine what cue will be used to remind him or her to begin the task. This could include having a parent or teacher (or sibling or friend) provide the reminder, setting some kind of alarm, or using a naturally occurring event as the cue.
3. At the point when the child is expected to begin the task, make sure he or she does so promptly, reinforcing the child when he or she does not require additional cues beyond those he or she built into the plan.
4. Gradually fade the supervision.

This skill also lends itself to an incentive system to reinforce practicing the skill successfully. The child could earn points, for instance, for starting the task on time, with points redeemable for small rewards.

(cont.)

117

TABLE 6.5. *(cont.)*

<u>Vignette</u>

Lisa, age 9, had a very difficult time starting her homework promptly at the time her parents set for her (right after dinner). Her parents decided they needed to teach this as a skill. Every day when she came home from school, her mother sat down with her and they made out a homework plan (see Form 5.3, the Daily Homework Planner *on p. 201 in the Appendix). Lisa made a list of all her assignments and she wrote down when she would start each one. She was allowed to build in a break for one TV show. When it was time for her to start her homework, her mother pulled out the* Homework Planner *and asked Lisa to take a look at it. Lisa then got out the first assignment and her mother made sure she got off to a good start before she left to do other things. In the beginning, Lisa's mother praised her for following her schedule and when she completed each activity. As time went on, Lisa was able to make her schedule and follow it all by herself.*

<u>Keys to success</u>

1. Be diligent about consistency during the initial "habit-building" period. When this intervention breaks down, it's usually because the system wasn't followed consistently in the first few weeks.
2. Fade the cuing system gradually and do not hesitate to restart it if task initiation begins to fall off.
3. If the child is not quickly successful, institute an incentive system.

TABLE 6.6. Planning

Description of skill

The ability to create a roadmap to reach a goal or to complete a task. It also involves being able to make decisions about what's important to focus on and what's not important.

Environmental modifications

By modifying the environment, the necessity for the youngster to rely on his or her own planning skills is reduced. Modifications might include:

- Have the adult provide a plan or a schedule for the child to follow.
- Use scoring rubrics when giving students assignments.
- Break long-term projects into clearly defined subtasks and attach deadlines to each subtask (many teachers incorporate this into their long-term project requirements).
- Create a template (see *Long-Term Projects* teaching routine in Chapter 5).

Teaching the skill

The best way to teach children to plan is to walk them through the planning process many times with multiple kinds of tasks, gradually turning over the process to the youngsters by asking questions that prompt them to think about how to make a plan. In the early stages, the questions will need to prompt each step ("What do you have to do first?" "What do you have to do next?"). As youngsters become more experienced with this, the prompts can be more general (e.g., "OK, let's make a list of all the things you have to do to complete this project"; "Now let's organize those tasks in the order in which you need to do them").

Using the analogy of the roadmap may be an effective way to help students think about what planning requires. Using this analogy, have the youngsters identify the destination (or goal). Then have them visualize the path they need to take to reach the destination. With younger children, giving them a planning sheet that actually looks like a roadmap may facilitate the process.

Vignette

Tom, an eighth grader, had a bad habit of leaving projects until the last minute and then having no idea what he had to do to complete the assignment. This created a great deal of tension at home as he experienced meltdowns as deadlines approached. His mother finally decided to intervene. Using a weekly progress report, she arranged with the school to be notified directly when long-term projects were assigned. Then she sat down with Tom to draw up a plan for each assignment using the Long-Term Project-Planning Sheet (see Form 5.7 on p. 206 in the Appendix). The first time they used it, Tom had to write a report on a dangerous sea animal. She helped Tom brainstorm topics and identify all the materials he needed to complete the project. Then they took a calendar and, as they planned each step, wrote down deadlines on the calendar. Then they placed the calendar in a prominent place in the kitchen so Tom could check it easily each day. Since they used a form and calendar to complete the planning process, Tom's mother could gradually turn the process over to him. Eventually, she was able to remind him to do the planning, but he could do the rest on his own.

Keys to success

1. Ensure that the plan is detailed enough for the steps to be specific and behaviorally defined.
2. Ensure that the plan is realistic and that the child hasn't attempted to take on too much.
3. If the child is struggling, provide a specific time line and check in with him or her at those times.

TABLE 6.7. Organization

Description of skill

The ability to design and maintain systems for keeping track of information or materials.

Environmental modifications

One basic environmental modification presents itself for this particular executive skill: Youngsters who lack organizational capacity need to be given organizational schemes to work with. For this to work successfully, two other components need to be built in: Children need to be cued to use the organizational scheme, and they need to be reinforced for doing so. Examples of the kinds of organizational schemes children might be taught to use are

- Room-cleaning schemes. This can be facilitated by giving children plastic bins labeled for the possessions that are to be stored in each one.
- A system for organizing a backpack, such as specific pockets for lunch, permission slips, or money.
- A system for organizing schoolwork, such as using different colored folders to distinguish completed assignments from work not yet done.
- A system for organizing the student's desk, either at home or at school.

Many parents and teachers are quite adept at creating organizational schemes for youngsters. Where the process breaks down is the degree of supervision required to ensure that the child actually uses the scheme on a day-in, day-out basis. We also recommend adding a powerful reinforcer to ensure that the youngster uses the scheme. We know of a mother of a middle school student who threatened to send to Goodwill any clothes her son left lying on his bedroom floor. Although we generally recommend using positive reinforcement, we have to admit that this was a powerful incentive for this youngster to keep his bedroom clean.

Teaching the skill

For youngsters with genuinely weak organizational skills, teaching this skill is a long-term proposition. For the youngest of children, an important prerequisite is the ability to separate or categorize (see how this is incorporated into the *Desk-Cleaning Routine* in Chapter 5). Once youngsters have learned this skill, then we recommend teaching them to become organized by giving them lots of different organizational schemes for different aspects of their lives and having them overlearn those schemes (via cuing, practice, and reinforcement). As they internalize the schemes, the cuing and reinforcement can be faded.

Giving youngsters a variety of organizational systems will provide them with common templates on which they can draw when they begin to develop their own systems. Once they have internalized the schemes provided to them, new tasks can be introduced and they can be asked to hypothesize new organizational schemes to fit those tasks. At first they will need assistance in doing this, but they should be encouraged to look upon the process as a problem to be solved for which creativity may be required. For youngsters with weak organizational skills, working with a coach, as described in Chapter 7, may be an effective intervention.

Vignettes

Josh, a fifth grader, had the messiest desk in his class. He lost papers all the time, and it took him way longer than anyone else to locate his work materials. His teacher, Mr. Carroll, used to let a month go by, then keep him in from recess to get his desk clean. Josh hated missing recess, and his teacher hated nagging him. Finally, Mr. Carroll decided there might be a better way. Although Josh was the worst, there were others in the class that had messy desks too, so Mr. Carroll decided that Friday afternoons would be desk-cleaning time. Those who had clean desks could get a jump-start on their homework

(cont.)

TABLE 6.7. *(cont.)*

for the weekend. He brainstormed with the class what steps students need to go through to clean their desks. They created a checklist (see Form 5.5, Desk-Cleaning Checklist, on p. 203 in the Appendix). Now every Friday Mr. Carroll quickly checks each desk and decides who needs to use the checklist to clean their desk.

Joan, a ninth grader, was forever losing worksheets and assignments. She tended to work slowly and, at the end of class, was still taking notes and rushing to write down her assignments and gather her things. As a result, she tended to stuff papers into her notebooks or folded them into her books without paying close attention to where she was storing them. This led to lost assignments, and it was having a big impact on her grades. She decided to work with a coach to improve her organizational skills (coaching is described in Chapter 7). Their first step was to analyze what she was doing now. Joan was using a large three-ring binder separated by subject with an envelope at the beginning of each section. Although she tried to place worksheets, assignments, notes, and so on into the appropriate section, in her rush at the end of class she often failed to do this. Together, she and her coach designed a simpler system. They decided Joan would use two folders—one green and one red. In the green folder, she was to place all the assignments she was given for all subjects. As she finished each assignment, she immediately placed it in the red folder, ready to hand in. At the beginning of each class, Joan pulled out both folders. She looked in the red folder to see if she had any assignments to hand in for that class, and she set the green folder on her desk in preparation for any assignments she might get that period. Every day when she met with her coach, they discussed whether she remembered to follow her organizational scheme. Joan remarked that she had felt a little funny at first, with two brightly colored folders on her desk, but she felt better when a friend of hers noticed what she was doing, asked her about it, and liked the idea so much she began using the same system herself.

Keys to success

1. Develop a system of organization with the child that is relatively simple and has a visual or written template to follow.
2. Build in time daily (or whatever the time frame designated) for the child to use the organizational strategy.
3. Monitor the system regularly. By regularly, this usually means *daily* for a long time before the monitoring can safely be faded.

TABLE 6.8. Time Management

Description of skill

The capacity to estimate how much time one has, how to allocate, and how to stay within time limits and deadlines.

Environmental modifications

Refer also to the suggestions under *Sustained Attention* (Table 6.4) and *Task Initiation* (Table 6.5). Time management is a higher-level executive skill that includes a number of components such as the ability to follow and make a schedule, to plan and organize, to estimate how long it takes to complete tasks, and to monitor progress in the course of completing tasks to ensure that one is "on schedule." This is a very difficult skill for many to learn because youngsters with poor time management skills tend to lack not only the ability to estimate how long it takes to do something but also lack a sense of *time urgency*—or the concept that something needs to be completed in a timely and efficient manner. These skills are needed both to ensure that students don't wait until the last minute and to ensure that they work efficiently once they begin a task. For youngsters who have weak time management skills, environmental modifications to reduce the negative effects of this weakness might include the following:

- Give youngsters a schedule to follow and prompt them at each step of the way.
- Impose time limits and provide reminders for how much time is left.
- Use cuing devices such as clocks, bells, or alarms.

Teaching the skill

Youngsters need a number of prerequisite skills in order to manage time effectively, including the ability to tell time, the ability to make and follow a schedule, and the ability to estimate how long it takes to do something. We've already discussed making schedules in Table 6.6. Learning to estimate involves (1) helping the youngster understand what the task involves (e.g., the steps required to complete the task and how long it will take to do each step), and (2) a realistic sense of what the likely distracters, diversions, and roadblocks are and how they will impact the schedule and time estimates. Teaching estimation, therefore, involves having the youngster make a plan to accomplish the task and guess how long each step will take. The youngster can then compare his or her estimates to the actual time required. If the two numbers don't match, then some discussion of the factors that contributed to the mismatch should take place. If the youngster finds him- or herself susceptible to distractions, then he or she should put in place a strategy to minimize distractions.

The easiest way to instill a sense of time urgency is to make the end point of the task a critical event or meaningful consequence. For instance, if a child is slow to get ready to go to school in the morning and has to walk to school because he or she misses the bus, then this consequence may be salient enough for the child to get ready more quickly. Some parents effectively use access to fun activities to build in this sense of time urgency: for example, the budding hockey star may find it easier to get homework done quickly if he or she knows that if it's not done before hockey practice, he or she doesn't get to go.

As with the other more complex executive skills, coaching is often an effective process for helping youngsters acquire good time management skills.

Vignette

Fred, an 11th grader, was constantly getting work done at the last minute or asking teachers to give him extensions for due dates. He had perfected the art of believable excuses—way beyond "the dog ate it" or "my computer crashed"—and he was considering writing a book on the subject that he thought would be a best seller among his classmates. However, his teachers were losing patience with him, and he finally decided he needed to bite the bullet. One of his teachers offered to act as his coach to help him tackle the problem.

(cont.)

TABLE 6.8 *(cont.)*

They decided that the first step was for him to learn to better estimate how long it would take to do things. Each day they looked at his homework for the day and Fred wrote down how long he thought it would take him to do each task. When he did his homework, he wrote down the actual start and finish time and compared reality with his estimate. Slowly Fred learned that it usually took him at least 25% longer to complete a task than he thought it would. With this knowledge, he began to improve his estimates and to plan his time better. In the process of working on this skill, he and his coach also realized that Fred had a tendency to commit himself to too many activities. He was involved in several after-school clubs, was on the Student Council, and had a part-time job on the weekends. With his coach's help, Fred made some hard decisions about which activities he wanted to continue with and which he should give up. This was not easy for him, but he found it did make a difference. When his dad showed up late for dinner for the fourth night in a row, Fred kidded him about how he needed to learn to "say no." His dad looked startled, and it dawned on Fred that he was learning a life skill that might help him long after he finished school.

Keys to success

1. Help the student develop time awareness by practicing time estimation with class or homework assignments.
2. Bring the student's attention to time regularly and use the Premack Principle to reinforce this (first work, then fun stuff).

TABLE 6.9. Goal-Directed Persistence

Description of skill

The capacity to have a goal, follow through to the completion of the goal, and not be put off by or distracted by competing interests.

Environmental modifications

The environmental modifications for this executive skill are similar to those for *Time Management* (Table 6.8). For youngsters with weak goal-directed persistence, accommodating this weakness means that rather than rely on them to establish a goal and persist to achieve the goal, adults both give them goals and prompt them to keep on track. For this to work effectively, the goals set should be ones that the youngsters have some motivation to work toward. Involving them as full partners in establishing those goals is often the best way to do this. If they have trouble establishing goals for themselves, giving them choices for what they might want to work toward may make this easier for them.

An effective way to enhance a youngster's motivation to work toward a goal is to make that goal as real and as visible to the youngster as possible. For instance, if parents want their son to go to college, they might arrange for him to visit likely colleges early in high school so that he has a concrete impression of the college experience that he can draw on as he continues in high school. A 16-year-old who wants to save money to buy a car might tack a picture of a car on his or her bedroom wall or a bulletin board by his or her desk.

Ideally, the goal should be in sight. With younger children, this means setting goals so that the time it takes to reach the goal is quite short. With older youngsters, ways can be found both to keep the goal in sight (like the car on the bulletin board). Giving a youngster feedback about his or her progress in achieving the goal can help the youngster persist in his or her efforts. For instance, the youngster saving for a car might keep a bar graph showing how much money he or she has saved so far. Revisiting the goal frequently, for example, in the course of the coaching process, can also keep the goal real for the youngster.

Teaching the skill

The most effective procedure we know of for teaching goal-directed persistence is to use a coaching process. Chapter 7 outlines this process.

Vignette

Ever since she could remember, Amy wanted to be an archaeologist when she grew up. She read every book she could get her hands on. She was particularly interested in the Native American cultures of the Southwest, and she spoke quite knowledgeably on the subject to anyone who would listen. By the time she began her sophomore year in high school, however, Amy realized that the grades she was earning were probably not good enough to get her to her goal. When her parents tried to talk with her about this, she just got angry: "What does algebra have to do with archaeology?" she fumed. "And why do I have to read The Red Badge of Courage? *It has nothing to do with what I'm interested in." Amy's parents, in frustration, took her to see a counselor. Once they'd established some trust between them and Amy began to value the counselor's opinion, the counselor began talking with her about her long-term goals. She persuaded her that although it seemed as though a lot of high school requirements had nothing to do with what she wanted to do when she grew up, getting poor grades would close a lot of doors for her. Amy was a smart girl, and good grades came easily to her when she was younger. She realized it would not take too much more effort for her to bring her grades up if she set that as a goal. Together, she and her counselor set some marking period goals. They talked about each subject and what grade Amy thought she could earn in that subject. They also talked about what she would have to do differently to earn those grades. Although she saw the counselor only once a week, she agreed to e-mail her counselor*

(cont.)

TABLE 6.9. *(cont.)*

every day outlining her study plan. The next day, she would let her counselor know whether she had followed her plan. After about 6 weeks, she felt that she was following the routine enough so she could cut back to weekly check-ins with her counselor. By the end of the marking period, she had brought up all her grades and was close to making the honor roll. When she discussed her report card with her counselor, she set as her goal making the honor roll by the end of the next marking period. Her parents also arranged for the family to take a vacation to Arizona. They planned to visit both some archaeological sites and the campus of Arizona State University—a college with a strong archaeology program that Amy wanted to check out.

Keys to success
1. If the goal is in the distant future, establish shorter-term, interim objectives so that the student can see concrete progress.
2. Remember that the time horizon of the student is likely to be considerably shorter than that of the adult, and adjust accordingly.

TABLE 6.10. Flexibility

Description of skill

The ability to revise plans in the face of obstacles, setbacks, new information, or mistakes, or an ability to changing conditions.

Environmental modifications

For youngsters who tend to be inflexible, environmental modifications primarily involve reducing the demands for flexibility. These may include:

- Reducing novelty. This can be done (1) by advance familiarization with places, schedules, or activities through the use of "dry runs" or rehearsals; (2) preteaching or giving the youngster the opportunity to preview material to be presented; (3) providing advance warning, such as cuing the child in advance of transitions; (4) systematic, gradual exposure to new situations; or (5) participation in rule-based social groups to provide social experiences in a more structured setting.
- Modifying the nature of the task. This can be done by (1) decreasing the speed, volume, or complexity of information presentation; (2) breaking down tasks into component parts; (3) adapting open-ended tasks to make them more closed ended; or (4) providing the students with templates or rubrics to follow.
- Helping youngsters reframe the situation. This can be done by labeling problem situations to reduce uncertainty or creating social stories to help children understand and cope. Social stories are tailored to the individual child's unique situation and incorporate a description of the problem in a way the child identifies with easily as well as a solution or coping strategy that the child can use.
- Increasing the level of support around the task. This can be done by (1) offering high frequency of reassurance or reinforcement, (2) step-by-step assistance in working through difficult problems, (3) graded exposure or guided mastery, (4) close contact at transition times, or (5) cuing the child to use coping strategies (see below).

Teaching the skill

The first step in teaching youngsters to become more flexible is to help them understand what inflexibility is and then to teach them to recognize when they feel themselves being inflexible. You might explain to a child, for instance, that being inflexible means thinking there's only one right answer or only one path to a solution when, in fact, there are typically several right answers or several paths. Individuals who lack flexibility tend, without even realizing it, to create an imaginary scenario of what they expect to happen and then to rehearse that scenario in their minds until it becomes a "mental set." When reality doesn't match that mental set, the outcome for those individuals is confusion, agitation, anger, or frustration. This might be analogous to how you might feel upon learning that the plane you expected to take to New York is actually going to Chicago—and you only discover this as the plane is touching down at O'Hare Airport!

Once youngsters are able to recognize inflexibility in themselves, the next step is to teach them coping strategies for managing the emotions and the situation. Teaching coping strategies, of course, involves modeling, practice, feedback, and generalization to real settings, with cues to prompt the youngster to use the strategy until it is internalized. Coping strategies might include:

- Giving youngsters plans or rules for managing specific situations that arise frequently and cuing them to follow the plans or rules until they become internalized.
- Helping students develop "default" strategies they can fall back on.
- Providing scripts that can be used in problem situations (this could be incorporated into social stories, described above).

(cont.)

TABLE 6.10. *(cont.)*

- Teaching relaxation strategies, thought-stopping, or attention diversion strategies (e.g., through the use of visual imagery).
- Teaching youngsters the concept of an "error factor" to reduce absolutist thinking. For instance, some children become very upset in sports situations when an umpire or referee makes a call that they think is wrong. Preparing children in advance for this by letting them know that those officiating games are "allowed" to make mistakes may reduce unhappiness when perceived bad calls are made.

An approach that combines teaching students to recognize inflexibility and learning coping strategies involves the use of "5-point scales." This is described in more detail in the section dealing with *Emotional Control* (Table 6.3). A number of the teaching routines in Chapter 5 address problems with flexibility.

Vignette

Jeff, age 10, was a creature of habit. He struggled with transitions to new situations and always had difficulty in the first few weeks of each new grade until he became familiar with the schedule and with his teachers' expectations. In fourth grade he continued to struggle even after 2 1/2 months. His teacher followed a schedule, but she expected increased independence on the part of her students, so they had to be more flexible in accommodating to their work production and the time they needed for help. This was very frustrating to Jeff. Each day when he came into school he expected that his teacher would do reading and language arts before recess and math right after recess. He struggled a bit with writing but looked forward to math because it was clear-cut; black and white. When writing spilled over into math time Jeff got very upset and sometimes refused to finish. To help Jeff with this, his teacher started to check in with him every morning. If the language arts material for the day looked complex and she felt that it may run into math time, she presented an altered schedule that would help him to "reset" his expectations. She also set the criteria for his completion of language arts work, and when this was done he had the option of starting some math. Over time, she planned to work with Jeff on developing a personal schedule so that he learned to estimate how much time his work would take. The goal for Jeff was to learn that an "estimate" is just that, and hence that schedules—and Jeff—needed to have some flexibility.

Keys to success

1. Add changes into the student's day/schedule. Initially do this with the addition of preferred activities with warnings and then, as the child adjusts, without warning. As the child gets used to this, move on to "neutral" and then less preferred activities and reward the child for managing the change without major difficulty. Tell the child beforehand that this is the pattern that will be followed.
2. "Inoculate" the child to change by presenting it in small doses.

TABLE 6.11. Metacognition

Description of skill

The ability to stand back and take a bird's-eye view of oneself in a situation. It is also an ability to observe how you problem solve and includes self-monitoring and self-evaluative skills (e.g., asking yourself, "How am I doing?" or "How did I do?").

Environmental modifications

These are designed to prompt children to use analytic skills to assess how they are performing assigned tasks. They include:

- Embedding questions designed to elicit metacognition into daily classroom instruction. Here are some examples of questions teachers might ask: "How did you solve that problem?" "Can you think of another way of doing that?" "What can you do to help remember that information?" See other sample questions in Table 4.3 on p. 57.
- Building error monitoring into task assignments (e.g., by requiring children to show that they have checked their work when doing math computations or by having them fill out proofreading checklists before handing in writing assignments).
- Giving children assignments requiring them to use metacognitive skills. For example, they could be asked to give themselves a grade on an assignment and to explain why they feel they deserve that grade.
- Using scoring rubrics to define what a quality product or assignment will include.

Teaching the skill

Metacognition is such a broad executive skill that one specific set of procedures for teaching the skill cannot be identified. Examples of teaching procedures might include the following:

- Have children develop error-monitoring checklists and then prompt them to use them, gradually fading the prompts.
- Teach children a set of questions to ask themselves when confronted with problem situations. Here are some questions they might ask: (1) "What is my problem (problem definition)?" (2) "What is my plan (solution strategy)?" (3) "Am I following my plan (self-monitoring prompt)?" (4) "How did I do (self-evaluation)?" These questions could be written in a list form and publicly displayed. Parents or teachers could then prompt the child to go through the set of questions when problem situations arise.
- Teach the child to ask him- or herself specific questions in problem situations, with the questions tailored to the specific problem. For instance, if a child tends to invade other children's personal space resulting in annoyance or rejection, he or she might be taught to ask him- or herself, "Did I get too close?" and to move away from the other child if the answer is "yes." He or she might also be taught that the definition of "too close" is "if the child is closer to me than two shoe lengths."
- As with many of the skills described so far, the procedure for teaching the child to use metacognitive skills includes (1) defining the skill to be learned, (2) listing the steps the child goes through in using the skill, (3) practicing the skill in a controlled setting, (4) cuing the child to use the skill in the natural environment, (5) reinforcing the child for using the skill either verbally or through the use of an incentive system, and (6) fading the cues and reinforcement.

Vignettes

Sam, in second grade, made many mistakes in math. On math computation, he often failed to note the operation that he was supposed to perform; as a result he often added when he should have been subtracting or vice versa. His teacher kept handing papers back with low grades and reminders to "Watch the signs!" When his performance did not improve, she decided that he needed to learn a

(cont.)

TABLE 6.11. *(cont.)*

procedure that would help him to do the problems correctly. She taught him to say to himself as he began each problem, "Am I adding or subtracting?" She and Sam practiced this a lot; she also sent a note home to his parents so that they could use the same process to help him with his homework. With enough practice, he began making a lot fewer mistakes.

Joe, in fifth grade, also tended to make careless mistakes in math, but his problem was different from Sam's. When Joe had to solve multistep problems, he stopped after the first step and gave that number as his answer. His teacher also taught him a procedure. Now, when he has to solve a math problem, he first figures out each step and then writes down a notation for that step as a reminder. For instance, he's given the problem, "If you buy 5 candy bars for 60 cents each, how much change should you get back from 5 dollars?" His teacher taught him to say, "First I multiple 5 times 60 cents," then write down an M for multiply on his paper. Then he says, "I take that number and subtract it from 5 dollars," writing an S for subtraction on the paper. As he completes each step, he crosses out the letter describing that step.

Keys to success

1. Since the heart of metacognition is self-monitoring and self-evaluation, ensure that the student is an active participant in the checking and evaluation process. This requires that the process be simple enough for the student to understand and eventually apply independently.
2. Encourage or cue the student to use the strategy or think about the monitoring/evaluation process prior to beginning the task and acknowledge strategy use with specific praise or a reward and by explaining what the strategy use accomplished.

CHAPTER 7

Coaching Students
with Executive Skills Deficits

In previous chapters, we described several general intervention strategies for enhancing executive skills or minimizing the negative effect of weak executive skills, as well as specific interventions targeted to individual executive skills deficits and everyday problem situations that arise because of executive skills weaknesses. Through our work with children and adults who had traumatic brain injuries we were well aware of the relationship between frontal lobe injuries and deficits in executive skills even in so-called "minor" head injuries. We also recognized executive skills weaknesses in many of the children with attention disorders with whom we worked.

Coaching grew out of an intervention that we originally described as mentoring. We recommended this strategy for some of the students with attention-deficit/hyperactivity disorder (ADHD) and learning disabilities we worked with who needed help organizing and remembering their materials and structuring their time. Hallowell and Ratey, in their book *Driven to Distraction* (1994), briefly described a coach as an "individual standing on the sideline with a whistle around his or her neck barking out encouragement, directions, and reminders to the player in the game. . . . Mainly, the coach keeps the player focused on the task at hand and offers encouragement along the way" (p. 226). We liked this notion of a coach and felt that it fit well with our idea of mentoring.

At around this time, Russell Barkley (1997) presented his theory on the relationship between executive skills weaknesses and ADHD. A third element contributing to our coaching model emerged from the behavioral literature on correspondence training. Defined by Paniagua (1992, p. 227) as a chain of behaviors that, "include a verbalization or report about past or future behavior and the corresponding nonverbal behavior," one aspect of correspondence training involves making a verbal commitment to engage in a behavior at some later point. This verbal commitment increases the likelihood that the behavior will actually take place.

By weaving these various elements together into a system, we felt that the coaching process could be an effective intervention for students. We developed each stage of the coaching model to correspond to an aspect of executive skills and incorporated correspondence training by including in each coaching session a verbal and written commitment on the part of the student to carry out the objectives for that day. Thus, coaching was developed as a systematic training process that initially provides a person with access to the executive skills he or she needs to accomplish a goal. The process serves, via the coach and the associated documentation, as a "lend-lease frontal lobe," available on a temporary basis as the student develops his or her own executive skills.

Coaching embodies some unique aspects. To succeed, the process requires the student's willing and active participation at each step, a factor not always in evidence in intervention strategies with children. Related to this, coaching is continuously collaborative, encouraging the child or adolescent to make decisions and choices. The process is designed to be managed by the student and the coach, independent of parental supervision. This can serve to defuse conflict or criticism that may have developed around performance issues.

As an intervention, coaching operates simultaneously at three levels. The first level involves the accomplishment of a task or set of tasks satisfying some performance standard in the student's environment (e.g., parent or teacher expectations, grades). The second level continuously draws a connection between day-to-day (or minute-to-minute) tasks and the student's longer-term goal, satisfying the student's own sense of accomplishment and efficacy. The third level teaches, on a daily basis, a set of executive skills and over time gradually fades the coach's role and increases the student's active use of these skills. In addition, the coach encourages the development of new goals and the student's use of executive skills to achieve these goals, thus promoting generalization and transfer.

Given the active and collaborative nature of the approach, coaching is most successful with students who are willing and active participants and who have made a commitment to change. Hence, when reluctant students have been "talked into" or, worse yet, coerced into participation in the coaching process, it is unlikely to succeed. At the same time, we have found that when younger students are approached with a problem that the adult has noted ("Caitlin, it seems that completion of your math work in class is a problem. Would you be willing to work with me on a plan to complete your work?"), they usually are willing to participate in the coaching process. When individual coaching is the intervention of choice with late middle school and high school students, the choice of participation and who will be the coach rests largely with them.

In terms of teaching executive skills, by virtue of his or her role as a "lend–lease frontal lobe," the coach has a unique opportunity to assess the student's executive skills strengths and weaknesses. From this assessment the coach can determine which skill or skills represent the most significant impediment to achieving the goal, and gradually fading his or her support in these areas to promote transfer and generalization of skills.

The coaching process begins with the assumption that a student is having difficulty achieving a particular goal that is important to him or her and/or an adult. Hence, the purpose of coaching is to work on and accomplish some goal or goals. Coaching with children of all ages is a two-step process. In Step 1, the student selects a goal or set of goals he or she wants to work on. In Step 2, the student identifies tasks he or she needs to do on a daily basis in order to achieve his or her goal. The two stages of coaching are briefly summarized in Table 7.1.

While students all have an individual pattern of executive skills strengths and weaknesses, the coaching process is flexible enough to enable students to work from their own unique profile, both "shoring up" weak executive skills and taking advantage of executive skills strengths to work around or compensate for the areas of weakness. Table 7.2 describes how the elements of the coaching process can address each executive skill domain.

COACHING OVERVIEW

Step 1: Conduct a Goal-Setting Session

The first step in coaching is to help the student identify a goal he or she would like to work on. The goal selected will depend in part on the age and developmental level of the child, in part on the child's interests, and in part on what parents or teachers think are important behaviors for the youngster to work on.

With elementary-age children, the goal will generally be something that can be accomplished on a daily basis. For instance, one student may decide he or she wants to work on getting daily assignments completed on time. Another student may decide he or she wants to work on raising his or her hand before speaking in class.

TABLE 7.1. Overview of the Coaching Process

Step 1: Conduct a goal-setting session.

This session should include three components:

1. Setting a goal. This may be a daily, weekly, or marking period goal, depending on the age and developmental level of the student. Older high school students should be encouraged to set a long-term goal that addresses their plans following high school completion.
2. Identifying potential obstacles to achieving the goal and ways to overcome the obstacles.
3. Writing a plan for achieving the goal.

Step 2: Hold daily coaching sessions.

The purpose of the daily coaching session is to make a plan for the day. There is some flexibility in how daily coaching sessions are conducted, but in general, the first part of the session is spent reviewing the previous day's plan and the second part is spent designing the plan for the current day. This may include asking the student the following questions:

1. Did you complete the tasks you said you were going to do yesterday?
2. Were you satisfied with the amount of time and effort you put into those tasks?
3. What do you have to do for today? [Make a list]
4. When are you going to do each of the tasks you've identified?
5. Are there other activities or responsibilities you have to work around in order to complete today's plan?
6. Are there long-term projects or exams coming up that we need to begin planning for?
7. Given how things are going, are you on target to achieve the goal you set in Step 1?

TABLE 7.2. How Coaching Facilitates Executive Skills Development

Executive skill	How coaching addresses this skill
Goal-directed persistence	This is the overarching purpose of coaching: By engaging in the process students learn how to make and achieve long-term goals.
Planning	• In goal-setting session, student is asked to develop a plan to achieve desired goals. • In daily coaching session, student makes daily homework plan.
Metacognition	• In goal-setting session, student is asked to consider potential obstacles to achieving goals and to think of ways to overcome obstacles. • In daily coaching session, student is asked to assess how well the previous day's plan went and how to improve likelihood of success in the future if problems arose.
Time management	This skill is developed through making daily plans; coach has student estimate how long each task will take and to think about how to fit in non-school related activities, such as jobs, sports, etc., along with homework, including studying for tests and working on long-term assignments.
Organization	Coach can use homework such as writing assignments or notebook checks to help student develop organizational schemes.
Emotional control	Student learns to manage frustration associated with obstacles to goal attainment or to successful completion of daily plans.
Flexibility	Students with weaknesses in this skill practice it not only through managing obstacles and changes in plans as they arise, but, if necessary through the coach working with them on how to handle assignments, such as open-ended tasks, that are often difficult for inflexible students.
Task initiation	By asking students to specify when a given task will be started, the coach helps the student follow through on plans and begin tasks in a timely fashion.
Sustained attention	By asking students to commit to a daily plan, student learns that tasks need to be seen through to completion.
Working memory	Asking students to make a daily plan prompts them to remember all the work they have to do, including both daily homework and long-term assignments. The daily plan itself serves to jog the student's memory to ensure all work is completed as scheduled.
Response inhibition	By making a plan and learning to set and meet daily goals, students are also learning to avoid the temptation of setting aside work to engage impulsively in whatever fun activities arise to compete with work.

By the middle school level, some students are ready to set somewhat longer-term goals. We often recommend that students at this age set marking period goals. For instance, an eighth grader may decide he or she wants to work toward earning a B in science, his or her most difficult subject. Or a seventh-grade boy for whom discipline is an issue may decide he wants to finish the marking period having earned no more than three after-school detentions for talking back to his teacher.

At the high school level, we still recommend that students set marking period goals, but many students are also ready to begin thinking more long term. For example, the coach may help them establish a goal related to what they want to do after high school.

The developmental differences in coaching involve not only how long term the goals may be, but also whether the process is chosen by the adult or by the student. Whereas in high school we believe it works best as a student choice, at the elementary and middle school level, coaching can be integrated into the student's daily schedule (e.g., during time in the resource room or a study hall). In all cases, we recommend that the coach be someone the student enjoys working with, and that whenever possible we recommend that the choice of a coach be given to students themselves.

Once the goal is established, this first phase of the coaching process includes a discussion of the potential obstacles students may encounter in their efforts to reach their goal as well as the steps they may need to follow in order to achieve the goals. Coaches may be able to help students identify supports both within the school and at home they can draw on to help them reach their goals. For instance, if an elementary student is working on completing work in a timely fashion, he or she may arrange to do some of his or her seatwork in a quiet corner of the classroom or in the resource room in order to minimize distractions. At the middle school level, students may decide to stay after school and participate in an after-school homework club if they have set as a goal getting homework handed in on time and completed. For high school students who may identify earning certain grades in specific subjects, coaches should discuss with them what grades they earned in the past and what they think they need to do differently in order to reach their goals.

While this discussion takes place at the beginning of the coaching process, the goal set is frequently referred back to as coaching gets under way. This is particularly important if the executive skill being worked on relates to "goal-directed persistence," since it's very important to keep the long-term goal clearly in mind (or in working memory) as the process unfolds.

Step 2: Hold Daily Coaching Sessions

Once a coaching relationship has been established and a goal set, then students and coaches meet on a daily basis to make plans for what they will work on that day to bring them closer to their goal and to assess how successful their efforts have been. Generally, this is done by having the coach ask the student a series of questions designed to help him or her formulate a plan for the day. When the coaching process is under way, the first part of the session involves reviewing the plan made the day before and evaluating the student's success at following the plan. Then a new plan is drawn up. In so doing, the coach helps the student think about the plan in depth, both to identify all the necessary steps and to anticipate what problems the student may encounter in following the plan.

For many daily plans, there are two key ingredients that students need to include. First, they need to specify exactly *what* they are going to do. Second, they need to specify *when* they are going to do each task. There is a body of research (e.g., Paniagua, 1992) that demonstrates that making a public commitment to perform a task vastly increases the likelihood that the individual making the commitment will actually carry out the task. Correspondence involves the agreement between a verbal description of what one will do and actually doing it; that is, *correspondence* between what I say and what I do. One aspect of correspondence training involves a verbal statement that one will engage in a behavior at some later point. This verbal commitment, particularly if public, increases the likelihood that the behavior will actually take place.

The specific plan the coach and student draw up, of course, depends on the goal being worked on. Again, with younger children, since goals tend to be quite simple and precise, the plan may be easy to formulate and quite straightforward. For instance, if the goal of an elementary-age child is to remember to bring home at the end of the day the materials needed for homework, then the coach and student together might make a list of what those materials are and the child can agree to check off the list as he or she gathers the appropriate materials to put in his or her backpack at the end of the day. For this particular example, holding the coaching session at the end of the day will make it easier for the coach and child to make their plan and for the child to follow through.

With older students, since the goals tend to be longer term and more complex, the plan is likely to be somewhat more complicated. For instance, with high school students who are trying to develop good planning/organization or time management skills, developing the plan may include both reviewing with the student the assignments that are due the next day as well as any upcoming tests or long-term projects or papers the student needs to be working on. Part of the planning process might include breaking down long-term assignments into subtasks and assigning due dates to each subtask, as well as determining what needs to get done by the next day. Then the student makes a list of everything he or she needs to do before tomorrow and identifies when each task will be done. It may be the job of the coach to push the student to be as specific as possible, both in terms of what the student will do and when he or she will do it. For instance, if the student says he or she will study for his or her science test right after supper, the coach may want to down pin the student both in terms of how much time he or she plans to spend studying but also *how* he or she intends to study (e.g., by making flash cards of key terms, writing out questions on index cards with answers on the back, going back and highlighting notes, or creating a graphic to visually organize notes). This degree of specificity will be more essential with some students than others.

While it is the job of a coach to help students plan, problem solve, and evaluate their efforts, it is also the job of the coach to act as a mentor and cheerleader. For some students, having an adult cheering them on as they aim for goals that seem lofty to them can make the difference between success and failure. Coaches can also act as go-betweens or mediators when students encounter problems related to the coaching goals.

The applications of coaching are many and varied, but to give the reader a sense of how the process works, let's create a dialogue that might take place between a high school student and his coach. Let's assume the following conversation takes place in the first daily coaching session.

COACH: Joe, you've set as a goal for the marking period to bring your English grade up to a B. This will take some work on your part, since last marking period you got a C. Do you remember what you said you were going to try to do differently to improve your grade?

JOE: Yes, I'm going to study for my weekly vocabulary tests, I'm going to stay on top of my reading assignments, and I'm not going to leave papers until the night before they're due so I'll have time to edit and revise.

COACH: Excellent. All good ideas. If you can follow through on them, I'm sure your grade will improve. The coaching we're going to do should help you do this. What we will do when we get together every day is to make a plan for the day that will help you reach your goal. So why don't we begin by taking a look at what's coming up in English. Do you have anything due for that class tomorrow?

JOE: Yes, I'm supposed to read the first chapter of *Lord of the Flies*.

COACH: Anything else—any study questions to answer or reader response you have to write?

JOE: No, except we're supposed to keep an eye out for something that might *foreshadow* later events in the book.

COACH: How are you planning on doing that?

JOE: Well, Ms. Hancock told us we should look for tensions between characters that might be likely to get worse as the book goes along. Or maybe look for things that are important to characters or maybe personality traits or character flaws that might get them in trouble . . . things like that.

COACH: Sounds good. How are you going to keep track of your ideas?

JOE: I have my own paperback copy of the book, so I thought I would put the letter F in the margin by each detail that might be foreshadowing.

COACH: Sounds like a good plan. When do you think you'll be able to do this assignment?

JOE: I was planning on doing it in my seventh-period study hall.

COACH: Do you think that will give you enough time?

JOE: I think so, but if not, I can finish it after basketball practice and just before dinner.

COACH: OK. Let's talk about upcoming English assignments. What's on the horizon?

JOE: (*consulting his agenda book*) I have a vocabulary test on Thursday, and by next Monday I have to have read the first three chapters of *Lord of the Flies* and write a reader response.

COACH: So you have 3 nights before the vocabulary test. Have you thought about how you might use the time to study?

JOE: (*a little sheepishly*) I wasn't even going to think about this until Wednesday night. That's a big improvement over last marking period, when I didn't study at all!

COACH: There's actually some good research to show that spreading out studying into several short sessions is a more effective way to learn material than to cram the night before. But tell you what, let's use this week as a baseline. Why don't you plan to study the night before and we'll look at your quiz grade. Then we can decide if you might want to try a different approach next week. . . . So, what's your plan with reading the rest of *Lord of the Flies* and writing the response?

JOE: I thought I'd read the other two chapters on Saturday and write the response on Sunday night.

COACH: Let me make a suggestion. You may want to look at how many pages you'll have to read for the second and third chapters and divide the total by the number of days you have left until Sunday. If you can read a little each day, it'll be easier to stay on top of the reading. Maybe you can take advantage of little pieces of time like in study hall or while you're waiting for dinner.

JOE: I like that idea. I'm a slow reader so what's gotten me in trouble before is not allowing enough time to do all the reading *and* write the response.

COACH: You've left the paper until the night before it's due. One of your strategies was not to do that.

JOE: Oh, I meant leaving *big* papers until the last minute. This is just a little thing I should be able to whip off in less than an hour.

COACH: Do you need help thinking about how to write your paper?

JOE: Nah, I'm good at that. I did lousy before because I'd only do half the reading and then I'd try to fake it. If I can get the reading done, the paper should be a piece of cake.

COACH: All right. I think we have a plan for today. With the work you have set for English, do you think you'll be able to fit in your other homework, too?

JOE: I think so. English has always been bad because I don't like it and I kept putting it off. If this'll help me stay on top of the work, I should be fine.

COACH: Great! I think this process will work well for you. You're off to a good start. Writing down assignments and keeping track of what's due when is an important part of the process and it seems like you do that well.

JOE: Yeah, well having enough teachers drum into me the importance of writing things down finally got through to me. See you tomorrow, "Coach"!

The next session would begin by having the coach and Joe pull out the plan they created the day before and review it to see whether Joe followed the plan—both in terms of doing what he said he was going to do and in terms of the time commitment. If Joe deviates from the plan, then the coach would be wise to explore with Joe what got in the way and to keep those obstacles in mind when making future plans. Then a new plan is drawn up. The coach should again review with Joe both immediate assignments and the long-term assignments he also needs to stay on top of. Each day the coach should ask Joe whether he's been assigned anything long term that he needs to think about. And even though Joe's goal pertains only to bringing up his English grade, it will be important for Joe not to lose sight of the work he has to do for other classes, as well as other obligations such as basketball games, any job he may have, or any family obligations that will take time away from studying and reaching his goal.

Initially, coaching sessions should occur daily. As can be seen from the above scenario, it does not need to be a long process and can fairly quickly become a routine. Consistency is critical, however, both for the student and the coach. Over time, daily coaching sessions can be gradually faded, first by having the student and coach meet every other day, perhaps, and eventually reducing the sessions to once every week or every other week. If the fading procedure leads to the student's failure to stay on track, then sessions need to be scheduled more frequently again.

The most effective coaching we have seen takes place in the school with an adult the youngster knows well and is comfortable with acting as the student's coach. We have known students who have selected other students to act as their coaches, but when this is done, we recommend that an adult serve as "back-up coach" to monitor the process and step in when problems arise.

We also think the process has group applications. Many middle schools and high schools assign students to "advisor groups" that meet daily or frequently (e.g., during homeroom period). With some modifications, including group instruction in how the coaching process works and a training period to get the process up and running, we think group coaching can be successful, either by pairing students in a peer coaching model (see below) or by having the teacher lead the group in setting individual goals and reporting back to the group students' success in meeting those goals. Group applications, of course, have the added advantage of enabling the classroom teacher to address the needs of many students without having to allot individual time to each one.

BUILDING COACHING INTO THE STUDENT'S EDUCATIONAL PROGRAM

We see coaching as having a number of applications in the school setting. For students of almost any age struggling with independent work management, effective use of time, or self-regulation of behavior, coaching may play a role, and we have seen it used effectively as a component of individualized education plan (IEP) and 504 plans. In terms of establishing a coaching intervention in school there are a number of considerations:

• Does the problem to be solved lend itself to a coaching intervention? A reading problem would not lend itself to coaching but in most cases, an executive skills problem would.

• Is the student a willing and active participant? With all students, but particularly those in late middle and high school, the viability of coaching depends on the student's active choice to be involved.

• Can a good fit between student and coach be achieved? With older students, we ask them to select their coach from among school staff. Younger children are more open to suggestions but they must indicate comfort with the person who will be their coach.

• Does the prospective coach understand the commitment? Once the process has begun, the actual daily contact ranges from 5 to 10 minutes. Despite this seemingly brief encounter, consistency is key and if the coach becomes haphazard in his or her commitment, the intervention rapidly fails. Similarly, if the student's immediate success is taken as a sign that the problem has resolved and coaching can be discontinued, the problem frequently resurfaces.

• Is there a plan for gradually fading the intervention along with continuing measurement of the target behavior to ensure that the student has acquired the skill and can manage independently? When coaching is chosen as an intervention, we recommend that a written plan including the participants, goals chosen, type and frequency of contact, and recording format be developed and that a brief summary of the results be included. Such a record is an important component of an IEP or 504 plan and can help to determine whether this is a viable intervention strategy.

EVIDENCE OF COACHING EFFICACY

In the process of developing our coaching model, we conducted a pilot study at a high school in New Hampshire. Six student volunteers were solicited, and individual coaches from the guidance and special education departments were trained in the process. One student dropped out, but the remaining five were coached for two marking periods. To evaluate efficacy, we conducted exit interviews with coaches and looked at student report card grades in the year before coaching occurred and during the two marking periods in which the process was conducted. Table 7.3 demonstrates that grades improved during the time coaching was in place.

There have also been a number of published studies that provide evidence of the success of coaching with a variety of age groups and outcome measures. Merriman and Codding (2008) demonstrated the efficacy of our coaching model for ADHD students at a high school level. Dependent variables in their study included homework completion and accuracy in math. The coaching procedure incorporated goal setting and self-monitoring as well as a fading procedure. The authors reported improvements in work completed ranging from 60 to 88% over baseline. By the end of the intervention, the students involved were completing at least 80% of their assignments with at least 80% accuracy. Significantly, all of the students involved rated the treatment package as highly acceptable.

Schultz, Evans, and Serpell (2009) investigated the use of a mentoring model with middle school students diagnosed with ADHD that focused on organization, self-monitoring, and social skills. They concluded from their findings that this model significantly reduced

TABLE 7.3. Impact of Coaching on Report Card Grades

% grades earned	B or better	C	D
Before coaching	19	61	19
During coaching	63	32	5

or delayed the onset of failure experiences in sixth- and seventh-grade students. While they did not use our model for coaching, the results suggest that a coaching type of intervention can significantly impact the school performance of a population that is at particular risk for executive skills weaknesses.

Peer Coaching

While our original coaching model (Dawson & Guare, 1998) was predicated on using an adult as coach, we had also considered the possibility of peers as coaches. Subsequent clinical and research work by ourselves and others suggests that peer coaching may be a powerful application of the coaching process to assist with the development of executive skills. Peer coaching has a number of advantages. Peers are available to act as models for each other throughout the day since they are part of the natural school environment. With peers as coaches, large numbers of children can be served while the labor intensity of the model is significantly reduced. Peer coaching is potentially a very effective model for learning the skills, particularly with reciprocal coaching, since each child is both coach and "player" or teacher and student. Moreover, as a classwide intervention, peer coaching means that an awareness of executive skills pervades the environment.

Based on some recent research that used our original coaching model to develop a peer coaching intervention, we envision at least two ways in which peer coaching could be used. One of these is at a classwide level involving all students acting as reciprocal coaches for each other. The second involves a more targeted intervention using selected students as coaches to work with other students who evidence more significant executive skill weaknesses. A study by Plumer and Stoner (2005) provides an excellent example for both applications. The objective of their study was to assess the impact of two different types of peer coaching on the social behavior of targeted students with ADHD who evidenced social skills deficits. At the classwide level, they used the classwide peer tutoring model (CWPT), which involves what we have called reciprocal peer coaching. Significant positive effects on the behavior and academic performance of elementary school students with ADHD using CWPT have been documented (DuPaul, Ervin, Hook, & McGoey, 1998). Plumer and Stoner (2005) used the CWPT component with an academic task (spelling) but were interested in the impact that this intervention would have on the social behavior of the children diagnosed with ADHD. In the treatment phase of this study, the authors adapted our coaching model for use by selected peer coaches, who were chosen by teacher nomination on the basis of their high frequency of appropriate classroom behavior. These students received specific training for their coaching role with the targeted students. In this study, Plumer and Stoner found that the CWPT had positive effects on children's academic and social behaviors in the academic setting but improvements in social interactions did not generalize to recess and lunch. However, with the addition of the peer coaching component the ADHD students did show significant improvements in social interactions in the school social settings. The authors concluded that our coaching model can effectively be extended to young children using elementary-age peers who were provided with coach training and adult supervision.

Two models are relevant for classwide reciprocal peer coaching. As noted above, CWPT has been extensively evaluated and proven to be an effective model for academic improvement across elementary and middle school environments. CWPT has a number of demonstrated advantages including the following:

- The model can be implemented in any school district or classroom.
- It can be implemented at little or no cost using existing materials.
- Although it has been used for academics, success of the model has suggested it could be used with almost any subject matter, particularly behaviorally defined executive skills.
- The model has been effectively used with students as young as first grade and the effects were shown to last at least 3 years after students received the training.

For executive skills training, a second and perhaps even more relevant model has been described in the literature as classroomwide peer-assisted self-management training (CWPASM; Mitchum, Young, West, & Benyo, 2001). This model has particular appeal in the executive skills realm since it focuses on self-management of behavior, which is the heart of executive skill processes. The model teaches self-management strategies to students and uses peers as coaches to help one another work on specific behaviors and to oversee the accuracy of self-monitoring measures, keys to the success of this process. A study by Mitchum et al. (2001) using middle school students showed significant improvements in on-task behavior, appropriate attention-getting strategies, and acceptable social interactions between peers for a classroom as a whole and for targeted students who had particular difficulties in these areas. The authors cite additional research demonstrating the efficacy of this model for younger students.

For more intensive interventions corresponding to Tier 2 in an RTI model, we envision a model similar to the one used by Plumer and Stoner (2005) in their study. In this model, we envision that students with strengths in those particular executive skills that the target students were weak in would be nominated by teachers. In this case, the peer coach's role would have some similarities to the adult coach in our model. The steps involved in setting up a peer coaching program are listed in Table 7.4.

In sum, based on our own clinical experience and on the research and clinical experience of others working in the field, we understand peer coaching to be a viable, effective intervention for children with executive skills weaknesses. In fact, by virtue of the advantages it offers for modeling, transfer and generalization of skills, along with decreased labor intensity for adult staff, peer coaching may in some cases be the intervention of choice.

TABLE 7.4. Overview of the Peer Coaching Program

Step	Task
Step 1:	Design coaching process: • Define role and specific functions of peer coach. • Outline coaching process, including meeting times and steps to be followed in the coaching interaction. • Design forms to document coaching as well as record-keeping forms to track outcomes. • Specify how, when, and by whom coaches will be supervised.
Step 2:	Select peer coaches on basis of executive skill strengths and solicit willingness to participate.
Step 3:	Identify target students and determine which executive skills and which daily activities will be addressed through coaching (e.g., target skill: working memory; daily activity: remembering to hand in homework).
Step 4:	Meet with target students to explain coaching; invite them to participate and to identify specific goals and objectives. Include a discussion of possible incentives to be earned if this is judged necessary (for many students, coaching by itself is a successful intervention while others require rewards on top of the coaching).
Step 5:	Contact parents of both coaches and target students to explain the process and obtain permission to participate.
Step 6:	Conduct training sessions with coaches. Adult plays role of target student to assess peer coach's understanding of the process and their ability to follow the template.
Step 7:	Meet with target student and coach to discuss how the process will work. Adult models the target student's role with the target student observing while the peer coach undertakes the coaching role. Answer questions and clear up any confusion. Target student and adult exchange roles, with adult observing while peer coach and target student go through a practice run of the coaching process. Explain use of forms and record keeping.
Step 8:	When adult is satisfied that both students understand their role and has reinforced them for their effectiveness, coaching begins, with the teacher monitoring the first few sessions.
Step 9:	Evaluate the process and make any adjustments necessary.
Step 10:	Peer coach and target student follow the coaching schedule set up, with the adult checking in one to two times per week with the coach and the target student to ensure that the process is on track and being correctly followed. Arrange for regular communication with parents regarding efficacy of intervention.

CHAPTER 8

Executive Skills Interventions within a Response-to-Intervention Framework

Chapter 3 provides an introduction to RTI and how executive skills development can be facilitated within a three-tiered intervention model. The emphasis in that chapter was on assessment, while this chapter focuses on interventions. In Chapter 4, we described three general methodologies teachers can use to support executive skills development. Here, we apply these interventions to the three-tiered model.

THE UNIVERSAL LEVEL

The universal level encompasses systems-level or classroom-level supports directed at *all* students and designed to meet the needs of *most* students. As a place to start, we can ask, "What do classrooms look like in which teachers build in systems, supports, and instructional strategies to support executive skill development?" Table 8.1 answers this question in the form of a checklist that can be used to determine if the classroom provides reasonable supports for students with executive skill weaknesses.

As we have worked with students and teachers over the years, the question that arises more often than any other is this: At what point do we expect students to be able to use executive skills effectively on their own without the need for external supports? A corollary to this question (sometimes spoken and sometimes implied) is by providing external supports, such as cues, reminders, and step-by-step instructions, aren't we slowing down the process by which students acquire these skills? In other words, are we *enabling* students or making them dependent on adults?

We have several answers to these questions:

1. Adults who work with students need to keep in mind that executive skills take a *full two decades* or longer to become fully mature. This means that the typical student will need some degree of support through the 12th grade. Students with disabilities, as well as students who have been shown to lag behind their peers in executive skills development (e.g., through rating scales such as the BRIEF or through a more comprehensive evaluation process), will require more intensive support and for a longer period of time.

2. Our general rule of thumb is this: Provide just enough support for the student to be successful. The principle includes two components that are of equal weight: (1) just enough support and (2) for the student to be successful. Adults who work with children tend to make two kinds of mistakes. If teachers provide too much support, the child is successful but fails to develop the ability to perform the task independently. If they provide too little support, the child fails, and, again, never develops the ability to perform the task independently. In our experience, at least from middle school on, teachers tend to provide too little direct instruction, modeling, and support in executive skills rather than too much.

3. Supports should be faded gradually. This applies both to individual students and to whole classrooms. For instance, one support that might be provided for classrooms is supervision to ensure assignments are written down in assignment books. Teachers often provide this supervision at the beginning of the school year and then discontinue it after 4–6 weeks. They may warn students that this will occur, but in our experience they often discontinue the practice abruptly. We believe a more effective educational approach would be to continue to build in time at the end of class for students to write down assignments and to cue them to do so, with spot checks of individual students to ensure that they are using the time as intended. Building in a "buddy system," whereby students sitting next to each other are charged with checking each other's assignment book is another way to keep the system in place while fading direct teacher supervision.

4. When teachers want students to take more responsibility for tasks associated with executive skills, they should teach them how to do this rather than expecting them to suddenly produce the skills on their own. For instance, if the goal is for students to be able to break down long-term assignments into subtasks and timelines, students should be given a template for this and the skill should be modeled and monitored. A teaching routine for helping students develop this skill is included in Chapter 5.

5. Finally, we have found that elementary school teachers tend to assume if a child fails to exhibit a certain executive skill, it's because it has not yet developed in the child or because the child has not yet been taught the skill. Somewhere around late elementary or early middle school, many teachers seem to shift their perspective on the problem. They no longer view it as a *skill* deficit and begin to view it as a *motivational* deficit. This leads to the assumption that if a student fails to carry out a task for which an executive skill is needed (such as remembering to bring home at the end of the day all materials needed to complete homework assignments), it's because the student doesn't care or doesn't want to. This is all the more likely to happen when the majority of students in a class are able to use the executive skill successfully, so that the student who fails to employ that skill is doing so willfully or intentionally. There may be an element of truth to this, but if we look at executive skills

development as habit training, then the assumption should be that if the student is not using the skill independently at least 80% of the time, then the habit is not yet fully ingrained, and continued prompting and supervision will be necessary.

With this in mind, the checklist in Table 8.1 is applicable to classrooms at all grade levels, with the understanding that more support and supervision will likely be necessary at the younger grade levels while less support and supervision will be required at the upper grade levels.

As outlined in Chapter 4, there are three primary intervention strategies to support executive skill development in students: (1) environmental modification to match the student's environment to the level of executive skill development; (2) instructional strategies to teach students missing or insufficient skills; and (3) incentive systems to help motivate students to use skills that are effortful. Table 8.2 shows what these strategies might look like at each of the three intervention tiers. At the universal level, the emphasis is on whole-class supports, such as class-wide routines that handle homework collection, whole-class instruc-

TABLE 8.1. Checklist of Classroom Supports in Tier 1 Classrooms

Managing classroom assignments	Ensure students: • Start promptly. • Complete on time. • Hand in when done.
Managing homework	Ensure students: • Write down assignments in assignment book. • Understand assignments. • Bring home necessary materials to do homework. • Hand in assignments on time.
Managing materials	Ensure students: • Keep desks organized. • Keep notebooks organized. • Maintain organizational systems.
Planning/time management	Help students: • Break down long-term assignments into subtasks and timelines. • Follow timelines. • Make daily homework plans.
Behavior management	• Post classroom rules. • Review rules frequently. • Model and practice rule following.
Promoting problem solving/independence	• Build in choice or self-directed study in assignments. • Encourage goal setting. • Use conflict mediation. • Teach problem solving for both social and academic problems.

TABLE 8.2. Strategies for Executive Skills Development at Three Levels

Intervention Tier	Environmental modifications	Instructional supports	Motivational strategies
Tier 1: Universal Systems-level or classroom-level supports directed at *all* students and designed to meet the needs of *most* students	• Establish classroom routines to manage things such as using an assignment book, handing in homework, planning for long-term assignments, maintaining notebooks. • Teach classroom rules for behavior (post prominently, review regularly, and practice for mastery). • Set up schoolwide monitoring/feedback systems (such as Power School or TeacherEase).	Teach: • Study skills necessary to meet course requirements (e.g., how to study for tests, how to break down long-term assignments into subtasks and timelines). • Organizational/working memory skills (e.g., how to maintain an assignment book, how to organize notebooks, how to remember important things such as due dates, permission slips, etc.). • Homework skills—how to plan homework sessions, strategies for getting started, screening out distractions, persisting until completion, avoiding temptation, and problem solving.	• Use group contingencies to meet specific criteria. • Build in fun activities following effortful classroom tasks. • Make liberal use of effective praise targeted to executive skill development.
Tier 2: Targeted Somewhat more intensive interventions to meet the needs of the 10–15% of students for whom universal supports are insufficient	• Modify assignments to increase likelihood of success (shorten, build in choice, make more closed-ended). • Set up after-school homework clubs. • Provide weekly progress reports to inform parents of missing assignments, upcoming deadlines.	• Set up small-group coaching for at-risk students to teach them how to make and follow homework plans and provide closer monitoring to students with working memory deficits or planning or organizational problems. • Institute peer tutoring programs or train volunteer tutors. • Contact parents to develop a simple plan to address the problem (e.g., arranging for progress reports).	• Home–school incentive systems (daily or weekly report cards). • Require students to use free time or after-school time to complete unfinished work.

(cont.)

TABLE 8.2. *(cont.)*

Intervention Tier	Environmental modifications	Instructional supports	Motivational strategies
Tier 3: Intensive			
For the 1–7% of students with chronic and more severe problems	At this level, an effective intervention involves working collaboratively with parents, teachers, and students to develop an individual support plan.	Elements of an effective intensive intervention: • Target behavior is well defined and includes criteria for success. • Specific environmental modifications are identified. • The skill is explicitly taught, modeled, and rehearsed on a regular basis. • Someone is assigned to check in with the student at least daily. • The student is given a visual reminder of expectations. • The student's independent use of the skill is monitored over time so that progress can be measured.	

tion to teach students how to manage homework sessions, and whole-class incentives such as using fun activities as a reward for completion of effortful tasks.

THE TARGETED LEVEL

The targeted level, or Tier 2, is designed to meet the needs of the 10–15% of the student population for whom universal supports are insufficient. Tier 2 interventions fall into two categories for the most part. Either they are small-group interventions, such as an after-school homework club or group coaching, or they plug students into programs that the school has established to meet the needs of individual students. Examples of these kinds of programs are

- Peer tutoring programs or volunteer tutoring programs targeting at-risk students.
- Weekly progress reports sent to parents (often by the guidance office) informing them of how students performed in the past week on key indicators (behavior, grades on tests/quizzes, missing homework assignments).
- Home–school report cards that inform parents about students' performance with respect to target behaviors so that they can administer reinforcers at home.

A third kind of Tier 2 intervention is assignment modification to match the student's level of executive skill development to the class or homework assignment. This may be more labor-intensive for the classroom teacher because there is no universal modification that applies to all executive skill weaknesses. With practice, however, we believe teachers can quickly assess the needs of students and make accommodations accordingly. The most common assignment modifications that are of benefit to youngsters with executive skill weaknesses are depicted in Table 8.3.

TABLE 8.3. Modifying Assignments for Students with Executive Skills Deficits

Assignment modification	Example
Shorten assignment.	• Have student do odd-numbered math problems only. • Have student work on math homework for 15 minutes and then stop (may need supervision).
Build in breaks.	• Ask student to show teacher his or her work every 10 minutes. • Send student on an errand at the completion of a seatwork assignment.
Allow choice.	• Give students multiple ways to study spelling words—ask them to choose one or two ways. • Create a menu of homework assignments and allow students to choose the ones that fit their learning style.
Provide templates or additional structure.	• Provide partially completed outlines to assist with note taking. • Provide graphic organizers to help students write papers or study for tests.
Make tasks more closed-ended.	• Have student write each spelling word five times rather than use each word in a sentence. • Give student highlighted social studies text to help him or her locate answers to chapter questions.

THE INTENSIVE LEVEL

This level is reserved for the 1–7% of students with chronic or more severe problems. Interventions at this level are highly individualized and, to be most effective, usually involve a collaborative effort that includes parents, teachers, and the student in the intervention design. Because, presumably, Tier 2 interventions have failed for students at this level, we recommend beginning with a functional behavioral assessment (FBA) to help identify other factors besides executive skill weaknesses that might be making the problem resistant to change. It is beyond the scope of this book to address this assessment process, but readers are referred to another book in this series, *Conducting School-Based Functional Behavioral Assessments* by Steege and Watson (2009), for a detailed description of how FBAs are conducted.

Table 8.2 lists the critical elements of an effective intervention at the intensive level. Figure 8.1 provides an example of such an intervention for a student with significant executive skill weaknesses.

MAKING DECISIONS REGARDING ELIGIBILITY FOR TIER 2 INTERVENTION

As noted in Chapter 3, the first step in addressing executive skills weaknesses in students is to put in place an intervention in the regular classroom, set a goal, and monitor progress

Behaviors of concern: Mike forgets assignments, forgets to bring materials home, and forgets to hand in assignments. He also has trouble managing his time and breaking down long-term projects into subtasks and making and following timelines. Problems are severe enough that Mike has failed several classes and is in danger of not earning enough credits to pass for the year.

School's responsibility: To assign a coach to work with Mike on strategies to improve recall, organization, planning, and time management.

Coach's Responsibility: To meet with Mike for the last 15–20 minutes every day in order to (1) review all homework assignments, including daily homework, upcoming tests, and long-term projects or papers; (2) break down long-term assignments into subtasks and develop timelines; (3) create a study plan for tests; (4) make a homework plan for the day; and (5) monitor how well the plan is followed and track assignment completion. The coach will also check in with teachers at least weekly (on Friday) to track any missing assignments and to double-check long-term assignments. Coach will e-mail parents on Friday informing them of any missing assignments.

Teachers' responsibility: To provide baseline data to determine current level of performance (e.g., percent assignments handed in on time), and to make sure Mike has ample time to write down his assignments at end of day and/or make sure website homework postings are current and explicit. Teachers will also respond by noon on Friday to coach's request for feedback about missing assignments.

Parents' responsibility: Mike will be allowed to spend Friday evening and Saturday with friends as long as homework assignments for the week have been handed in. Criterion will be determined from baseline performance. Parents will download e-mail from coach on Friday and have a feedback session with Mike before weekend plans are made.

Mike's responsibility: Mike will attend coaching sessions consistently and will participate in setting goals and making plans for homework completion.

FIGURE 8.1. Sample intensive-level executive skills student support plan.

toward that goal. If the goal is not met, then the school problem-solving team should meet to assess whether the intervention can be refined or another classroom-based intervention can be designed to address the behavior of concern. If the consensus is that the problem behavior cannot be resolved without additional supports or resources, then the next step is to look at the array of Tier 2 interventions available and select the most appropriate one.

For example, let's consider a middle school student named Pedro who hands in his homework on average once a week. His teachers have put in place systems to ensure that students write down the homework assignment and have the appropriate materials in their backpack at the end of class. They also have a system for collecting homework that holds students accountable (e.g., they can't leave the classroom without handing in their work or giving their teacher a plan for getting their homework handed in). Even with these supports in place, Pedro's homework assignment completion rate continues to be abysmal. His home-room teacher calls Pedro's parents to discuss the team's concerns and to ask whether his parents can monitor homework completion from their end. His mother says this is difficult to do because she and Pedro's father both work long hours, and they are attempting to manage home routines of several children in the evening. Pedro's mother promises to try, but Pedro continues to hand in homework only infrequently. At this point, the problem is brought to the school's problem-solving team. The decision is made to enroll Pedro in the after-school homework club, a Tier 2 intervention. Pedro is expected to attend the club 4 days a week and to bring with him his assignment book and all necessary homework materials so that he can get his homework done in this supervised setting. The team, which includes Pedro's parents and Pedro himself, set a goal of 85% homework completion and the team agrees to meet again in 6 weeks to assess progress toward the goal. If Pedro has met the goal, then there will be a discussion about whether he continues to require the support of the after-school homework club or if it can be faded gradually (e.g., by having him come for fewer days or spend less time at each session). If Pedro has not met the agreed-upon goal, then the team considers whether additional elements can be added to the Tier 2 intervention to make it successful (e.g., by adding a reinforcer that his parents could provide), or if he needs more intensive support.

GUIDELINES FOR PROGRESS MONITORING

RTI is most vulnerable to misuse or shortfalls when it comes to progress monitoring. We have been in problem-solving team meetings where the team leader explains to parents, "Well, we'll try a few things and then we'll get back to you to let you know whether they worked or not." This, of course, raises many questions: *What exactly* are they trying? What is the *criterion for success*? and *How long* will you try the intervention before making a decision regarding its efficacy?

There are no hard-and-fast rules to answer any of these questions, but any school that implements a RTI model must make decisions about how success will be determined and at what point moving to a different tier (either up or down) is warranted. With respect to academic goals, it may be possible to identify precise cut-off scores (e.g., no less than 20% below grade-level benchmark norms for words read correctly per minute) that determine the success of an intervention. With behavioral goals, including executive skills, univer-sal standards for success are unlikely. Nonetheless, a problem-solving team responsible for designing and implementing an intervention to address an executive skill weakness should define all aspects of the intervention including: (1) the behavioral goal; (2) the exact nature of the intervention; (3) the length of time the intervention will be implemented; (4) the criterion for success; and (5) the measurement procedure. Form 8.1 "Progress Monitoring: Response to Intervention," can be used for this purpose (see p. 216 in the Appendix). Figure 8.2 shows how this form might be used for the case of Pedro described above. Figure 8.3 depicts the data from Figure 8.2 in graph form.

For RTI to reach maturity as an intervention model, it must be applicable to the wide variety of problems that lead students to fail or to fail to achieve to their potential. It must go beyond addressing deficits in basic academic skills at the elementary level to address academic and behavioral deficits from kindergarten through high school. We believe this chapter provides a format for doing this, not only for executive skill weaknesses, but for behavior problems more generally.

Student's Name: _Pedro_

Tier level	Intervention	Start date	Review date	Criterion for success	Measurement procedure	Outcome	Next step
1	Classwide monitoring system to ensure homework is written down; homework materials in backpack	10/15	11/12	85% homework handed in on time	Calculate percent homework handed in on time	Average for 4 weeks: 20% homework handed in on time	Contact parent
1	Monitoring system plus contact with parents; they agree to make sure homework is done	11/12	12/3	85% homework handed in on time	Calculate percent homework handed in on time	Average for 3 weeks: 50% homework handed in on time	Move to Tier 2
2	Assign Pedro to after-school homework club	12/3	1/21	85% homework handed in on time	Calculate percent homework handed in on time	Average for 6 weeks: 90%	Continue with homework club for 6 more weeks
2	Assign Pedro to after-school homework club	1/21	3/4	85% homework handed in on time	Calculate percent homework handed in on time	Average for 6 weeks: 90%	Fade homework club—3 days with a written homework plan for the 4th day

FIGURE 8.2. Progress monitoring: Response to intervention.

151

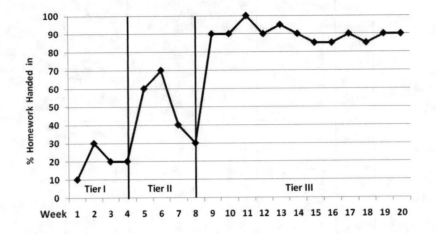

FIGURE 8.3. Homework completion rate at three intervention phases.

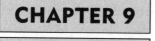

Applications to Specific Populations

As we have noted earlier, barring some catastrophic event, children are born with the capacity to develop executive skills. Within the brain of the newborn, these skills already exist as potential. The extent to which they develop depends on genetic and environmental factors, and we know that each child falls along a continuum with regard to his or her executive skills. Hence, children will have patterns of strengths and weaknesses. They may be poor at sustaining attention or initiating tasks, they may have mild problems with these skills, or they may be very good at them. For some, weaknesses in particular executive skills will be sufficient to interfere with daily living and school demands. In order to successfully meet these challenges, parents and teachers need to recognize the severity of the problem in the children with whom they work and adjust their efforts accordingly.

Children with executive skills weaknesses fall into at least three categories. We know that these weaknesses can occur in the absence of any currently recognized disorder or "diagnosis." Thus, one category comprises those children who have weaknesses in one or more executive skills in the absence of any other disorder or condition. A second category comprises those children who, by virtue of a certain condition or diagnosis, are likely to have a number of executive skills deficits. This category includes children with ADHD, children with autism spectrum disorders, and children with acquired brain injuries. The third category consists of children whose suspected executive skills weaknesses are confounded by other complex learning and/or social–emotional factors. We consider each of these categories in turn in the following sections.

EXECUTIVE SKILLS WEAKNESSES
IN THE ABSENCE OF A RECOGNIZED DISORDER

With respect to the first category, we know from clinical and research evidence that there are patterns of executive skills strengths and weaknesses in children (and adults) and that this is a normal and expected condition. For some children, the weaknesses will be minor and compensated for by their strengths. In other cases, the skill deficits will be sufficient to interfere with some aspect of work or problem solving. In our work, we've found some common or typical profiles of strengths and weaknesses. Children and adults who have strengths in some specific skills often show weaknesses in other particular skills and these patterns are predictable. For example, children with weaknesses in response inhibition also tend to have weaknesses in emotional control. They often act and emote without thinking, as likely to make an inappropriate comment as to fly into a rage with little provocation. Weaknesses in emotional control are also evident in children who are inflexible. Unexpected changes in plans can lead to behavioral and emotional meltdowns. Another pattern involves weaknesses with task initiation and sustained attention. Children with this type of pattern are slow to get started on school or homework and are likely to be distracted before it's done. Some of these children also have weaknesses in goal-directed persistence, and this combination leads to late or uncompleted work. However, we've seen evidence that if goal-directed persistence is relatively strong, that skill may compensate to some extent for weaknesses in task initiation and sustained attention. Thus, while work may be started late, it is more likely to be completed. Another typical combination in skills is seen in time management and planning/prioritization. Students who have these strengths rarely have difficulty managing long-term projects. However, if these skills are weak, students have difficulty determining both how and when to begin a project.

The objective in identifying strengths and weaknesses in a child's executive skills is to design and implement interventions to address those patterns. If we are able to do this, we can assist children in building the skills that they need to manage tasks or we can alter the environment to minimize problems associated with skill weaknesses.

The other key element in helping children with weaknesses in executive skills is the adult's understanding of his or her own pattern of executive skills. In working with children who have executive skill weaknesses, we have noted that a child's problem often seems more severe when the teacher and/or parent of that child has a very different pattern of strengths and weaknesses. If a particular set of skills comes easily to an adult, it is often difficult to understand how a child could struggle so significantly with the same set of skills. This lack of a "good fit" between adult and child increases the potential for conflict and makes it more difficult for the adult to see, through the child's eyes, what he or she is experiencing and what strategies might be of most help to him or her. When an adult has a clearer understanding about the nature of executive skills in general and his or her own pattern of strengths and weaknesses, it is easier to understand the child's behaviors and to develop intervention strategies that are a good match for the child. For an expanded discussion of "goodness of fit" see *Smart but Scattered* (Dawson & Guare, 2009).

DISORDERS THAT IMPACT EXECUTIVE FUNCTIONING

Attention-Deficit/Hyperactivity Disorder

Of the disorders and diagnoses implicated in executive skills deficits, ADHD is preeminent. While the other disorders considered below, such as acquired brain injury and autism spectrum disorders, typically involve more significant weaknesses in executive skills, the prevalence rates of ADHD in the population (conservatively 3 to 5%), indicate that there are a significant number of individuals with executive skill deficits.

What Is the Role That Executive Skills Play in ADHD?

In our opinion, Barkley (1997) made a comprehensive and compelling case that ADHD is fundamentally a deficit in executive skills. Since that time, a growing body of research has confirmed the role of executive skills in ADHD and delineated particular executive skill patterns in the subtypes of this disorder. Following Barkley's work, the development and publication of the BRIEF has provided a rich source of information about the role of executive skills in ADHD in everyday behaviors assessed by parents and teachers.

In a number of studies employing the BRIEF (Gioia et al., 2000), children identified with ADHD, in comparison to controls, were rated by parents as having significantly more executive problems than controls on all but one of the BRIEF scales. In the same study, using teacher ratings, children with ADHD had significantly more executive problems than did controls on all of the scales of the BRIEF teacher form. In addition, data on the BRIEF normative studies produced by Gioia et al. (2000), and by Guy, Isquith, and Gioia (2004) indicate significant differences in executive skills between children with ADHD and controls on parent, teacher, and self-report inventories of the BRIEF. Moreover, within the ADHD population, differences in executive skills are revealed between those with the inattention subtype and those with the combined subtype. Parent, teacher, and self-rating scales involving scales measuring Shift, Working Memory, Plan/Organize, Organization of Materials, and Task Completion differentiate the ADHD population from controls. Beyond that, the ADHD combined group have significantly more difficulties than the ADHD inattentive group on the Inhibit, Emotional Control, and Monitor Scales. Thus, on a well-validated scale of executive functions involving parent, teacher, and self-ratings, children with ADHD evidence significantly more executive skill weaknesses than controls and within the ADHD subtypes, differing executive skill profiles are observed.

Recent research has also looked at the relationship between cortical and subcortical structures and functions and executive skills. For example, Pliszka (2006) found that on a task involving behavioral inhibition, children with ADHD failed to activate regions in the left prefrontal and anterior cingulate cortex as determined on functional magnetic resonance imaging (fMRI). Durston et al. (2007) showed diminished activity in the cerebellum, prefrontal, and anterior cingulate cortex on fMRI data during tasks involving planning and behavioral adaptation to changing conditions. Shaw et al. (2007), using MRI scans, found significant delays in cortical maturation (thickness) in children with ADHD and noted that these delays were most marked in the lateral prefrontal cortex, which is involved in the executive skills of attention, behavioral inhibition, working memory, and evaluation of reward contingencies. This same study noted that children with ADHD had similar or earlier maturation in comparison to controls in primary motor areas, and the author speculated that this, in conjunction with delays in the prefrontal cortex development, may contribute to excess motor control problems. Finally, Plessen et al. (2006), on MRI data, found reduced connections between structures in the limbic system (hippocampus and amygdala) and the orbital frontal cortex of the brain and suggested that these reduced connections may be related to behavioral disinhibition in ADHD.

Thus, since Barkley's work in 1997, considerable evidence has accumulated in support of his position regarding ADHD as fundamentally one involving executive skills, and recent neuroscience research offers evidence that those brain regions suspected of involvement in ADHD and executive skills weaknesses do in fact show physical differences between ADHD and non-ADHD children. As we have suggested earlier, this, along with other neuroscience research, argues for early and sustained intervention for those children diagnosed with ADHD. In addition, accumulating evidence also suggests that differentiating among executive skills weaknesses in different subtypes of ADHD may allow for more targeted and effective intervention.

Autism Spectrum Disorders

Children on the autism spectrum have been identified as having executive skills deficits (Ozonoff & Griffith, 2000). For example, in a study of children with mixed disorders within the autism spectrum (Asperger's syndrome, autism, pervasive developmental disorder not otherwise specified) Gioia, Isquith, Guy, and Kenworthy (2000) report significant differences on the BRIEF when comparing these children to a control group. Significant deficits were noted in both the Metacognition and Behavioral Regulation Combined Scales reflecting global executive skill weaknesses. On the BRIEF self-report, Guy, Isquith, and Gioia (2004), note that most adolescents with Autism Spectrum Disorders reported difficulties on all of the BRIEF Scales except Inhibit.

In terms of more specific executive skills, children with high-functioning autism have been shown to have weaknesses in the metacognitive aspects of executive skills, specifically initiation and working memory. These skills were also noted to correlate with adaptive functioning in this population (Gilotty, Kenworthy, Sirian, Black, & Wagner, 2002). Other studies (e.g., Akshoomoff, 2005) have also noted the importance of metacognitive skills for children with autism spectrum disorders and have related deficits in these executive skills to problems with socialization and independent living. In terms of Asperger syndrome, Attwood (2007) cites a variety of studies confirming impairments in executive skills in children with this disorder. In addition to impairments in the broad range of executive and particularly metacognitive skills in children on the autism spectrum, clinical and research evidence points to particular difficulty in flexibility that we have defined as adaptability to changing conditions. In our clinical experience, emotional regulation is also a significant issue. Parents and teachers working with children on the autism spectrum experience, on a daily basis, the difficulty that these children have in dealing with transitions and unexpected changes. Because the weaknesses in executive skills for this population of children tend to be significant and sustained and thus have major implications for independence in socialization and activities of daily living, the need for ongoing, consistent, and long-term executive skills intervention is critical.

Acquired Brain Injury

Acquired brain injury involves an impairment in brain functioning as a result of either an external event such as head trauma or internal event such as tumor, infection, or stroke. In the case of a traumatic brain injury, impairments in executive skills are common and well documented as a result of the susceptibility of the frontal lobes to injury via acceleration and deceleration forces. For example, Gioia et al. (2000) noted that compared to matched controls, a group of children with severe traumatic brain injuries had significantly higher scores on a number of the Metacognition Scales of the BRIEF (e.g., Initiate, Plan/Organize, Working Memory) as well as on all scales of the Behavior Regulation Index. Moreover, children with severe traumatic brain injury had significantly higher scores on the Working Memory Scale than did children in the mild-to-moderate traumatic brain injury group and than in both control groups. Anderson, Jacobs, and Anderson (2008) cite research in traumatic brain injury implicating weaknesses in executive skills including inhibition, flexibility, planning, memory, and strategic learning. In a study by Yeates et al. (2004), deficits in the social outcomes of children with traumatic brain injury were related to deficits in specific neurocognitive skills, including executive functions. Deficits in executive skills as a result of severe traumatic brain injury are likely to persist over extended periods of time. Nadebaum, Anderson, and Catroppa (2007) found executive function deficits 5 years postinjury in children with traumatic brain injuries sustained before the age of 7.

In terms of etiology, children with acquired brain injury can represent a more diverse population than those with traumatic brain injury. For example, included in this population are children who have had brain tumors, strokes, infectious disease processes such as encephalitis, and neuronal migration disorders to name but a few. Not surprisingly, given the diversity of this population, no specific pattern of executive skill deficits has been identified although as studies increase and subpopulations are more clearly defined, it seems likely that some patterns will emerge. At this point, it is important to note that across these varying populations significant executive skills weaknesses have been identified. For example, studies by Mulhern et al. (2004), and Vaquero, Gomez, Quintero, Gonzalez-Rosa, and Marquez (2008) document the relationship between various types of brain tumors and executive functioning weaknesses in children. Anderson et al. (2008) cite their own research as well as that of others to indicate that the integrity of all brain systems is critical for adequate development of executive skills in early childhood. Thus, given the broad range of studies that have been conducted with children who have acquired brain injuries, it seems prudent to presume that a child with any type of significant acquired brain injury is likely to present with executive skill deficits until proven otherwise.

Other Populations

While we have not tried to exhaustively identify the populations for whom research suggests executive skills weaknesses, it is important to understand that beyond the groups identified above, executive skills weaknesses have been identified for children with obstructive sleep apnea, early treated phenylketonuria, and exposures to lead. Sleep disorders present some particularly interesting issues for executive skills weaknesses. More than 7% of children between the ages of 12 and 19 report symptoms associated with delayed sleep syndrome, a circadian disorder that results in difficulty falling asleep at normal bedtime hours (Pelayo, Thorpy, & Glovnsky, 1988). Thus, a significant portion of school-age children go to school in a sleep-deprived state. Children who are sleep deprived have been shown to have difficulty with initiating and persisting at tasks as well as problems with planning and goal-directed persistence on complex tasks.

In terms of other populations, recent research points to the impact of socioeconomic status (SES) of children on frontal lobe and executive skills development. For example, Nobel, Norman, and Farah (2005) found that SES has a disproportional impact on the development of left perisylvian/language and prefrontal/executive systems of the brain. Hackman and Farah (2009) report that SES is an important predictor of neurocognitive performance in the areas of language and executive skills. Thus, poverty may play a significant role in the delayed development of executive skills.

While these results involving children from low socioeconomic environments are certainly preliminary, for the other populations reported on above, for children with ADHD, children on the autism spectrum, and children with acquired brain injuries, there is definitive evidence of executive skills weaknesses. Moreover, in many of the studies reported these weaknesses are significant and have a clear impact on academics, activities of daily living, and social interactions. At the end of this chapter we summarize the specific information known about executive skills weaknesses in these populations to date and direct the reader to specific areas in this book relevant to those weaknesses.

Complicated Cases

The third category involves children who present with complicated issues of which executive skills may be one aspect. These cases manifest in at least two ways. Some children are initially referred for evaluation of executive skills with the presumption that weaknesses in such skills are at the heart of a problem, for example, that weaknesses in task initiation or goal-directed persistence result in poor work production. Thus, for example, we saw a male teenager with work production problems whose ratings on executive skills checklists by parents and teachers were well within the clinical range. A classroom observation confirmed problems with organization, task initiation, and goal-directed persistence. Observation also revealed little peer interaction and apparent disinterest in and lack of involvement in what appeared to be an active and engaging classroom. On questioning, parents and teachers indicated they had thought about depression but had assumed that the teenager's mood was reflective of school difficulties and the pressure he felt to perform. An informal academic survey revealed fair reading ability, a distaste for math, and some problems with written production. An interview with the young man indicated moderate depression of at least 6-months duration, currently exacerbated by a disruption in family relationships and rejection by a key peer in the classroom, as well as some long-standing discomfort with school. Further evaluation by a learning disabilities specialist revealed specific skill deficits in writing and math.

Initial intervention with this young man began with counseling and medication for the depression, a resolution of the teasing by the peer, and some individual help in writing and math. In the early stages, executive skills weaknesses were managed by external support from teaching staff with no emphasis on having the student learn and internalize these skills until he showed definite progress with the depression and academic weaknesses. Thus, a case that initially and reasonably appeared to be a set of problems related to executive skill deficits turned out, on further examination, to involve a more complex set of issues. In situations such as this where the initial presumption is one of executive skills weaknesses, certain findings might signal otherwise. Hence, it is important to understand that presenting problems such as decreased work output, missing deadlines, and losing materials can be influenced by variables other than or in addition to executive skills. Understanding what these variables are and the symptoms/behaviors by which they are manifest is critical to an accurate assessment and to an effective intervention. While in such cases a full evaluation may not be necessary, sufficient information needs to be gathered through observation, record review, checklists, and interviews to rule out learning, emotional, and psychosocial issues as principle factors or causes.

A second case we were involved in was that of a high school student who had been hospitalized on more than one occasion for suicide attempts. Although as a younger child she had been identified as having a speech–language handicap, in middle school the educational disability was changed to emotional disturbance. Whereas the school felt that depression accounted for her academic problems, her parents questioned this, citing examples of poor judgment on her part (racking up cell phone charges of several thousand dollars, for instance, and showing other poor problem-solving skills). On our evaluation, the BRIEF completed by her parents documented significant executive skills weaknesses, but so did other measures of executive skills, including measures of working memory and cognitive flexibility. We were particularly struck by her weak performance on a cognitive flexibility measure (the Animal Sorting subtest of the NEPSY-II), because it was consistent with her parent's report of the difficulty she had considering multiple options, seeing things from the perspective of others, and generating multiple possible solutions to problems. In this case, we felt that weak executive skills compounded her emotional problems and contributed to the risk of self-harm.

Complicated cases involving executive skills can also present at the outset as just that; complicated cases. Thus, children can be referred with evidence or a strong suspicion of cognitive-learning disabilities, attention disorders, and/or emotional–social problems. If no, or only limited, assessment has been completed prior to referral, then an evaluation sufficiently comprehensive to document functioning in these areas needs to be completed. Assessment of executive skills should be one component. The intended outcome of this comprehensive evaluation is a detailed, integrated picture of the child's strengths and weaknesses in these different areas and how they contribute to level of functioning and to the referral issue. For children beyond the early grades, evaluations have often been completed. In this case, rather than a comprehensive evaluation, the objective is to gather existing information, supplement for any missing evaluation pieces, and develop the same integrated picture. In either circumstance, children who manifest with complex problems (e.g., learning disabilities, emotional disorders) are already at risk for school failure. Executive skills weaknesses can compound the risk because of the role they play in work production and because as the child matures, there are fewer naturally occurring supports for these skills in the environment. Hence, it is important to assess these skills even when other significant problems have been identified. If executive weaknesses are identified, it is important to explain how these weaknesses interact with other problems, how they are likely to impact performance now and in the future, and what types of supports the student will need currently and in the coming grades to manage increasing demands.

IMPLICATIONS FOR INTERVENTION

For the populations of children described above with attention disorders, acquired brain injuries, and autism spectrum disorders, we know that they are likely to have particular patterns of executive skill weaknesses. Given the unique and varied nature of children, we would not suggest that these and only these skills will be impacted. Careful, individualized assessment of all executive skills is necessary for any child referred. Nonetheless, it is helpful to have a sense of those executive skills associated with conditions such as ADHD or traumatic brain injury or autism/Asperger diorder, because such knowledge can provide a framework for intervention and help the educator or clinician to be more efficient and accurate. To that end, we have attempted to summarize what is currently known or hypothesized about executive skills in relation to particular conditions and to point the reader in the direction of interventions for those executive skills.

- Children with ADHD, as a total group, show difficulties with working memory, flexibility, planning, organization, sustained attention, and task completion. Beyond that, those children who meet combined criteria (i.e., inattention and impulsivity) have greater difficulties than the inattentive group alone in self-regulation of affect, response inhibition and metacognition. In this volume, these specific skills are defined and addressed on pages 109, 113, and 128.
- For children on the autism spectrum who are in the category of high-functioning autism, particular difficulties have been noted with working memory, task initiation, and metacognition. We have addressed these skills on pages 111, 117, and 128. For children with Asperger syndrome, flexibility and emotional control are noted to be particular areas of weakness. These skills are addressed on pages 113 and 126.
- Within the population of children with acquired brain injuries, research involving children with severe traumatic brain injuries suggests weaknesses in the following skills: response inhibition, flexibility, planning, working memory task initiation and metacognition. Interventions for these skills are presented respectively on the following pages: 109, 111, 117, 119, 126, 128.

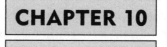

CHAPTER 10

Planning for Transitions

As students with executive skills weaknesses progress through school, they face a number of naturally occurring social, cultural, and institutional challenges that are based on our assumptions about how children change as they age. These assumptions can inadvertently exacerbate the student's executive skills weaknesses. For example, at the social and cultural level we expect, and in fact experience (for the most part), that children will become increasingly more independent with time. Hence, we also expect that they will be able to handle more complex school tasks and more responsibilities, and they will more effectively manage their own behavior. While we don't leave 6-year-old children alone, we are willing to do this for limited periods of time with children of 11 or 12 based on this assumption of improved self-management. Similarly, we don't expect 7- or 8-year olds to baby-sit without adult supervision, but we are willing to give this responsibility to a 14-year-old.

Schools also expect more independent application of previously learned skills, including improved time management, sustained attention to tasks, and self-regulation of behavior. In fact, consistent with this assumption, adults believe that as students age and progress through school, providing continued support may be a disservice to the student, undermining the development of independence and self-management, and creating a roadblock on their path to adulthood. How often have we heard from parents, teachers, and school administrators that students need to be more "responsible," "self-motivated," and "independent," and that if we support them or modify tasks they are expected to do, they will not learn to sufficiently manage on their own and will not be prepared for the next level of school development. Such supports are sometimes derogatively referred to as "babying" or "enabling" the student, or "dumbing down" the task.

We would argue that given what we know about executive skills development, students with weaknesses in these skills are in fact among the most vulnerable to underperformance and failure in school. Furthermore, these problems are directly related to the reduction of naturally occurring supports that earlier served as surrogate frontal lobes for these students. Further complicating the issue is the fact that as students age, underperformance or failure is more likely to be framed by adults as indicative of poor motivation, laziness, lack of responsibility, or some other behavioral (or moral) deficit, as opposed to a skill deficit within the child. Viewed in this way, underperformance or failure often has a volitional or "willful" component, and therefore will change only if the student is motivated to change and undergoes an "attitude" adjustment. The problem is that executive skills weaknesses often present as if they were motivationally driven; that is, as if the student could exercise voluntary control over them. However, Russell Barkley (1997) has elegantly explained why this is not the case when he points to executive skills weaknesses as biologically based motivational deficits.

Based on extensive research and clinical evidence, we know both that executive skills exist and executive skill weaknesses exist. We also know that weaknesses in executive skills can have a significant, adverse impact on school performance. Most important, we know that there are intervention models (e.g., coaching) that can facilitate the development of executive skills and lead to significant improvements in behavior and academic performance and that these interventions can be faded over time. We also know that such weaknesses cannot simply be "willed" away.

As a result of these developing trends and the naturally occurring drop-off in adult and institutional supports, students who may not have struggled significantly in earlier grades may now be exposed. This occurs because of the simultaneous increase in the level of performance demands and a decrease in the level of support. This exposure of executive skills weaknesses occurs not only in students as they move through school. We also have evidence that adults who may have performed well in one type of job situation may not be able to achieve the same level of performance or, in fact, may fail when they are promoted to another situation. This can happen when the new job demands a set of executive skills that were not previously important and thus there is an executive skill mismatch between the person and the job (Martin, Dawson, & Guare, 2007).

Prior to the time that the student passes through one of these transitional periods, executive skills weaknesses may not have been highly evident, because there has been sufficient support from parents and teachers or because there have been the naturally occurring classroom supports noted above, or because situational demands were low enough for the weaknesses to either not impact performance significantly or impact it only at the margins of performance. In these cases, adults may well assume or perhaps have been reassured that the child would "grow out of it." In the absence of significant difficulties prior to the transition, it may be easier for the receiving teachers to assume that the child is simply going through a temporary period of adjustment or that the performance drop-off is consistent with the developmental stage of the group as a whole. Thus, the assumption is that he or she will develop the skill or "grow out of" the problem. For those students who don't, it may be easier for teachers and administrators at the receiving level to see this as a responsibility or motivational issue. However, we would argue that students with seemingly benign profiles in the early grades who begin to struggle after a transition, have not suddenly become lazy, irresponsible, or unmotivated once they have moved to a more demanding level. Rather, the behavior and academic performance of the student has changed as a result of an acceleration of demands on executive skills and that the pejorative label applied to the student who appears to have the ability but does not perform is really a reflection of the social and cultural expectation that students will or should become more responsible.

Unfortunately, students so labeled can develop an aversion to school or to particular aspects or tasks within school and as a result look task avoidant, unmotivated, and irresponsible. Particularly in middle school and beyond, we have often seen a corresponding deterioration in behavior. This behavioral deterioration reflects the student's sense that it is better to appear defiant than "stupid." Since such defiance represents the natural challenge of adult authority by adolescents, this behavior is often both accepted and even encouraged by peers. Thus, not only does the student develop a strategy for avoiding failure but also for gathering some positive peer attention, and such a cycle can take on a life of its own. At the same time, these students may know and hear from others about how "bright" they are and about how they are not working up to their "potential," while having no understanding or explanation for why they are not succeeding. They may well chalk up the behavior to "stupidity" and/or they may accept the labels that they have heard so often from adults that they are "lazy," "unmotivated," or "don't work hard enough," and so on. These patterns of defiance and/or task avoidance can become self-fulfilling prophecies, as the failures continue without good explanation and as school becomes increasingly aversive. Not surprisingly, we have seen this type of situation lead to mood disorders such as anxiety and depression and to a longer-term loss of confidence and an inability to perform.

The difficulty is exacerbated by the fact that at times the student may actually rise to the occasion and perform adequately or even well, only confirming the adult's belief that the student has all the necessary skills but is choosing not to use them. The ability to succeed at times may come as a result of parental pressure, interest in a particular subject, desire to please a particular teacher, or some temporary good fit between the task and the student. The adult may conclude at that point, "I knew you could do it if you just really tried" and then decide that any future failure is the result of a lack of true effort. The student, continuing without an adequate explanation, may well accept this judgment, but that only leads to further frustration or discouragement. Potentially, the situation becomes one more reason not to try, because one success in a host of failures is only more frustrating and discouraging.

We know from our work on the impact of task effortfulness that for the child or adult with executive skills weaknesses, consistent sustained performance without significant help and support is very unlikely because it requires an ability to overcome, by sheer determination alone, what is in fact a skill deficit of the kind noted above as a biologically based motivational deficit. Hence, it is not a weakness that can simply be "willed" away any more than I can will away my inability to speak fluent French, even though, under the right circumstances, I might temporarily pass for or seem to have some fluency.

Given that students with executive skills weaknesses are particularly vulnerable during times of transition, what steps should be considered? If a decline in performance is evident and the student begins struggling at one of these major transition points, the following questions should be answered:

- Is there evidence that the student does better with supports, for example, homework help at home, or has he or she done better in the past with increased supports?
- What are the student's weakest and strongest subject areas and is there evidence of differential performance? In general, areas of strength are likely to require less in the way of executive skills.
- Does the weak academic area put a particular premium on executive skills? Language arts or English writing assignments require more in the way of executive skills as do responses to inferential questions or other types of inferential problem solving such as math where there may be a number of options to arrive at a solution.
- Is there a discrepancy between the student's ability and day-to-day production or achievement or a discrepancy between some measures (e.g., individual vs. group achievement tests) that might suggest that self-monitoring is a weakness?
- Does the student perform better when an adult is simply close by regardless of whether specific on-task cues are given?
- Is the area of weakness specifically related to an executive skill? For example, is the student struggling with organization of materials, time management, or planning/completion of projects?

Affirmative answers to any of these questions should lead to additional assessment of executive skills. We have provided questionnaires and structured interviews to facilitate this assessment, and we also recommend use of the BRIEF, which provides norm-referenced standards for evaluation of these skills at different ages.

We would urge school personnel and parents who are involved with students at these transition points to avoid the assumption that because a student moves up, a drop in performance must be related only to increased demands and more difficult content to which the student will adjust to in time. While this may be true, these performance problems often relate to greater demands on executive skills that until now have not been significantly taxed. This is especially true when students move from elementary to middle school, middle school to high school, and high school to college where executive skills demands are greatly increased and where teachers are often in the habit of attributing a drop in performance to the necessary learning curve and therefore to be expected, or to a student's lack of motivation or responsibility given the demand for increased effort.

Once a performance problem emerges, it is important to identify the specific subject, situation, and/or behavior where the breakdown is occurring and what supports might be available to address the problem (e.g., homework clubs, coaches, peer tutors). The parties involved (student, teacher, parent) should be given an explanation of what is happening in specific behavioral terms, the executive skill involved should be labeled, and the intervention most apt to address the problems should be identified. Whenever possible, the supports provided should not interfere with the student's ability to participate in the class and should be compatible with the instructor's teaching style and the expectations he or she has for his or her students. As noted earlier, the goal is to use the least amount of support necessary to help the student achieve successful performance and then to fade this help in a planned way so that the student gradually internalizes the executive skill. Keeping some type of data relative to the goal that has been set is important in determining whether the intervention is successful or whether modifications need to be made.

Finally, in the delivery of services for children in these transition periods, we would note a few cautions. Services should not be discontinued abruptly when the student experiences some initial success. Time-limited and short-term interventions assume that the student simply needed help in "getting over the hump." In fact, if the issue is one of executive skill weakness, more sustained intervention will be required to resolve the problem, and the criterion for discontinuing external supports should be evidence that the student has acquired the skill and now is able to manage independently. We would recommend that services rarely, if ever, be discontinued across the change of environments (e.g., one year to another, one school to another) since such a discontinuation assumes that the student has sufficiently mastered the skills to transfer to environments with new and unknown demands. If the student does show independent application of the skills and services are faded, performance should be passively monitored over one to two quarters to ensure that no decline has taken place. Whenever possible during these transition times, look for "goodness-of-fit" situations for the student. This might involve placement with teachers with instructional styles similar to those the student has been successful with in the past, greater organization and structure in the classroom, or a more active and hands-on teaching methodology. What constitutes the best fit depends on knowledge of both the student's strengths and weaknesses and executive skills profile along with that of the teacher's and the classroom situation.

Even with the most successful student following a normal developmental progression, it should be kept in mind that frontal lobes do not fully develop until individuals are in their early-to-mid-20s. For students with executive skills weaknesses significant enough to require intervention, full maturation may occur much later than that. It is our belief that with the kinds of strategies we have outlined in this book, teachers can have a significant impact on the development of these critical life skills. In so doing, they should take some satisfaction that not only have they helped students achieve success in school, but they have set them on a path to success in pursuits beyond high school.

Appendix
Reproducible Forms

167

Executive Skills Semistructured Interview—Parent Version

Many youngsters have problems in school or with homework not because they lack intelligence but because they have weak executive skills. These refer to the skills required to plan/prioritize (P) and carry out tasks, including time management (TM), working memory (WM), the ability to organize tasks and materials (O), task initiation (TI) and follow-through, flexibility (F), response inhibition (RI), emotional control (EC), sustained attention (SA), goal-directed persistence (GDP), and metacognition (M). I'm going to ask you some questions about _____ (fill in the child's name) to help us get a clearer understanding of his or her executive skills. Codes in parentheses refer to the specific executive skill measured by each item.

HOMEWORK. Which of the following areas, if any, does your child have difficulty with?

Item	Not a Problem	Notes
Understanding homework directions (M)		
Getting started on his or her own (TI)		
Being able to keep working despite distractions (SA)		
Asking for help when it's needed (M)		
Sticking with it long enough to complete it (SA, GDP)		
Making careless mistakes; failing to check work (M)		
Finishing the work on time (TM)		
Remembering to hand it in (WM)		

Are there some subjects or kinds of assignments your child is more likely than others to complete successfully?

More likely to be successful with . . .	Less likely to be successful with . . .

(cont.)

ORGANIZATION OF MATERIALS. Which of the following areas, if any, does your child have difficulty with?

Item	Not a Problem	Notes
Keeping notebooks and papers organized (O)		
Keeping desk tidy (O)		
Keeping belongings neat and in appropriate locations (e.g., gym clothes, coats, hats, mittens) (O)		
Keeping track of books, papers, pencils, etc. (O)		
Keeping backpack organized (O)		

LONG-TERM PROJECTS. Which of the following areas, if any, does your child have difficulty with?

Item	Not a Problem	Notes
Deciding on a topic (P)		
Breaking the assignment into smaller parts (P)		
Developing a timeline (P)		
Following a timeline (TM)		
Estimating how long it will take to finish (TM)		
Following directions carefully (WM, M)		
Proofreading or checking project to catch mistakes to make sure the rules were followed (M)		
Finishing the project by the deadline (GDP)		

(cont.)

REMEMBERING. Which of the following areas, if any, does your child have difficulty with?

Item	Not a Problem	Notes
Writing down assignments (WM		
Bringing home appropriate materials (e.g., books, workbooks, assignment book, worksheets, notices, permission slips, gym clothes) (WM)		
Bringing to school appropriate materials (see examples above) (WM)		
Remembering instructional sequences after normal instruction (e.g., long division, proper headings for papers) (WM)		
Remembering to perform chores or other household responsibilities (WM)		
Losing things within the home, yard, or neighborhood (WM)		

PROBLEM SOLVING. Which of the following areas, if any, does your child have difficulty with?

Item	Not a Problem	Notes
Recognizing that he or she has a problem (e.g., doesn't understand the directions) (M)		
Being able to think flexibly about the problem (e.g., not get stuck on one approach or solution) (F)		
Trying to solve the problem first on his or her own before going for help (M)		
Accessing appropriate resources to help him or her solve the problem (F)		
Evaluating his or her own performance to know whether the problem was solved successfully (M)		

(cont.)

SELF-CONTROL. Some youngsters have difficulty managing their behavior. Which of the following areas, if any, does your child have difficulty with?

Item	Not a Problem	Notes
Becoming easily upset (EC)		
Throwing temper tantrums (EC)		
Acting impulsively, either verbally or physically (e.g., provoking siblings) (RI)		
Interrupting others (RI)		
Difficulty waiting turn (RI)		

PARENTAL EXECUTIVE SKILLS. Do you see yourself as having challenges in any of the areas we've talked about? If so, in which areas?

Can you envision other problems with starting or following a plan? How or by whom could these problems be managed?

Executive Skills Semistructured Interview—Teacher Version

Many youngsters have problems in school or with homework not because they lack intelligence but because they have weak executive skills. These refer to the skills required to plan/prioritize (P) and carry out tasks, including time management (TM), working memory (WM), the ability to organize tasks and materials (O), task initiation (TI) and follow-through, flexibility (F), response inhibition (RI), emotional control (EC), sustained attention (SA), goal-directed persistence (GDP), and metacognition (M). I'm going to ask you some questions about _____ (fill in the child's name) to help us get a clearer understanding of his or her executive skills. Codes in parentheses refer to the specific executive skill measured by each item.

INDEPENDENT SEATWORK. Which of the following areas, if any, does the student have difficulty with?

Item	Not a Problem	Notes
Understanding task directions (M)		
Getting started on his or her own (TI)		
Being able to keep working despite distractions (SA)		
Asking for help when it's needed (M)		
Sticking with it long enough to complete it (SA, GDP)		
Making careless mistakes; failing to check work (M)		
Finishing the work on time (TM)		
Remembering to hand it in (WM)		

Are there some subjects or kinds of assignments that the student is more likely than others to complete successfully?

More likely to be successful with . . .	Less likely to be successful with . . .

(cont.)

ORGANIZATION OF MATERIALS. Which of the following areas, if any, does the student have difficulty with?

Item	Not a Problem	Notes
Keeping notebooks and papers organized (O)		
Keeping desk tidy (O)		
Keeping belongings neat and in appropriate locations (e.g., gym clothes, coats, hats, mittens) (O)		
Keeping track of books, papers, pencils, etc. (O)		
Keeping backpack organized (O)		

LONG-TERM PROJECTS. Which of the following areas, if any, does the student have difficulty with?

Item	Not a Problem	Notes
Deciding on a topic (P)		
Breaking the assignment into smaller parts (P)		
Developing a timeline (P)		
Following a timeline (TM)		
Estimating how long it will take to finish (TM)		
Following directions carefully (WM, M)		
Proofreading or checking project to catch mistakes to make sure the rules were followed (M)		
Finishing the project by the deadline (GDP)		

(cont.)

REMEMBERING. Which of the following areas, if any, does the student have difficulty with?

Item	Not a Problem	Notes
Writing down assignments (WM)		
Bringing home appropriate materials (e.g., books, workbooks, assignment book, worksheets, notices, permission slips, gym clothes) (WM)		
Bringing to school appropriate materials (see examples above) (WM)		
Remembering to follow classroom procedures (WM)		
Losing things in the classroom or other places in the school (e.g., lunchroom, gym, playground) (WM)		
Remembering instructional sequences after normal instruction (e.g., long division, proper headings for papers) (WM)		

PROBLEM SOLVING. Which of the following areas, if any, does the student have difficulty with?

Item	Not a Problem	Notes
Recognizing that he or she has a problem (e.g., doesn't understand the directions) (M)		
Being able to think flexibly about the problem (e.g., not get stuck on one approach or solution) (F)		
Trying to solve the problem first on his or her own before going for help (M)		
Accessing appropriate resources to help him or her solve the problem (F)		
Evaluating his or her own performance to know whether the problem was solved successfully (M)		

(cont.)

SELF-CONTROL. Some youngsters have difficulty managing their behavior. Which of the following areas, if any, does the student have difficulty with?

Item	Not a Problem	Notes
Becoming easily upset (EC)		
Throwing temper tantrums (EC)		
Acting impulsively, either verbally or physically (e.g., provoking siblings) (RI)		
Interrupting others (RI)		
Difficulty waiting turn (RI)		

CURRENT EFFORTS TO ADDRESS THE PROBLEM. Please identify the current strategies or interventions that are being used to address this student's problem areas and indicate how successful they are.

TEACHER EXECUTIVE SKILLS. Do you consider yourself as having challenges in any of the areas we've talked about? If so, will this have an impact on your ability to put in place interventions to address the student's problem areas?

Executive Skills Semistructured Interview—Student Version

I'm going to ask you some questions about situations related to your success as a student. All of these are situations in which you have to use planning and organizational skills in order to be successful. Some will be directly related to school, whereas other questions will touch on extracurricular activities, any job situations you've been in, and how you spend your leisure time.

HOMEWORK. I'm going to ask you some questions about homework and the kinds of problems kids sometimes have with homework. Please tell me if you think these are problems for you. I may ask you to give me examples of how you see it as a problem.

Item	Not a Problem	Notes
Getting started on homework. (TI) *Related questions:* What makes it hard? When is the best time to do homework? Are some subjects harder to start than others?		
Sticking with it long enough to get it done. (SA) *Related questions:* Is this worse with some subjects than others? What do you say to yourself that either leads you to give up or stick with it? Does the length of the assignment make a difference in your ability to complete it?		
Remembering assignments. (WM) *Related questions:* Do you have trouble remembering to write down assignments, bring home necessary materials, or hand in assignments? Do you lose things necessary to complete the task?		
Becoming distracted while doing homework. (SA) *Related questions:* What kinds of things distract you? Have you found places to study that minimize distractions? How do you handle the distractions when they come up?		
Having other things you'd rather do. (P, GDP) *Related questions:* Are there things you have trouble tearing yourself away from to do homework? Do you resent having homework or too much homework? Do you think there are other things in your life that are more important than homework?		

(cont.)

LONG-TERM PROJECTS. Now let's talk about long-term assignments. Which of the following, if any, are hard for you?

Item	Not a Problem	Notes
Choosing a topic (M)		
Breaking the assignment into smaller parts (P)		
Developing a timeline (P)		
Sticking with a timeline (TM)		
Estimating how long it will take to finish (TM)		
Following directions (e.g., Do you forget to do part of the assignment and lose points as a result?) (WM, M)		
Proofreading or checking your work to make sure you followed the rules and haven't made careless mistakes (M)		
Finishing the project by the deadline (GDP)		

STUDYING FOR TESTS. Here are some problems students sometimes have when studying for tests. Which ones, if any, are a problem for you?

Item	Not a Problem	Notes
Making yourself sit down and study (TI)		
Knowing what to study (M)		
Knowing how to study (M)		
Putting off studying/not studying at all (TM)		

(cont.)

STUDYING FOR TESTS. *(cont.)*

Item	Not a Problem	Notes
Taking breaks that are either too frequent or too long (SA)		
Giving up before you've studied enough (GDP)		
Memorizing the material (WM)		
Understanding the material (M)		

HOME CHORES/RESPONSIBILITIES. What kinds of chores, if any, do you have to do on a regular or irregular basis?

Chore	Regular (When do you do it?)	Occasional
1.		
2.		
3.		
4.		
5.		

What aspects of completing chores, if any, do you have trouble with?

Item	Not a Problem	Notes
Remembering to do them (WM)		
Doing them when you're supposed to (TI)		
Running out of steam before you're done (SA)		
Doing a sloppy job and getting in trouble for it (M)		

(cont.)

ORGANIZATIONAL SKILLS. Now I'm going to ask some questions about how organized you are. Tell me if you have problems with any of the following.

Item	Not a Problem	Notes
Keeping your bedroom neat (O)		
Keeping your notebooks organized (O)		
Keeping your backpack organized (O)		
Keeping your desk clean (O)		
Keeping your locker clean (O)		
Leaving your belongings all over the house (O)		
Leaving belongings other places (e.g., school, friend's houses, at work) (O)		
Losing or misplacing things (O)		

WORK/LEISURE TIME. Let's talk about how you spend your time when you're not in school. What kinds of extracurricular activities, if any, are you involved in? Do you have a job? How do you spend your leisure time?

Activity	Amount of time (approximate per day or week)
1.	
2.	
3.	
4.	
5.	
6.	
7.	

(cont.)

Here are some problems that students sometimes have with how they spend their spare time. Which ones, if any, are problems for you?

Item	Not a Problem	Notes
Spending too many hours at a job (TM)		
"Wasting" time (e.g., hanging out, playing computer/ video games, talking on the phone, time on Facebook, watching too much TV) (TM)		
Hanging out with kids who get in trouble (RI)		
Not getting enough sleep (RI)		
Spending money as soon as you get it (RI)		

LONG-TERM GOALS. Do you know what you want to do after high school?

Possible goals
1.
2.
3.
4.

Have you formulated a plan for reaching your goal(s)? If so, what is it?

(cont.)

What are some of the potential obstacles that might prevent you from reaching your goal(s)?

Potential obstacle	Ways to overcome the obstacle
1.	
2.	
3.	
4.	
5.	

If you have not yet identified a goal or developed a plan for reaching the goal, when do you think you will you do this?

Executive Skills Questionnaire for Parents/Teachers

Big problem	1
Moderate problem	2
Mild problem	3
Slight problem	4
No problem	5

Item   Score

1. Acts on impulse   _____
2. Gets in trouble for talking too much in class   _____
3. Says things without thinking   _____

                       TOTAL SCORE: _____

4. Says, "I'll do it later" and then forgets about it   _____
5. Forgets homework assignments or forgets to bring home needed materials   _____
6. Loses or misplaces belongings such as coats, mittens, sports equipment, etc.   _____

                       TOTAL SCORE: _____

7. Gets annoyed when homework is too hard or confusing or takes too long to finish   _____
8. Has a short fuse; easily frustrated   _____
9. Easily upset when things don't go as planned   _____

                       TOTAL SCORE: _____

10. Difficulty paying attention; easily distracted   _____
11. Runs out of steam before finishing homework or other tasks   _____
12. Problems sticking with schoolwork or chores until they are done   _____

                       TOTAL SCORE: _____

13. Puts off homework or chores until the last minute   _____
14. Difficulty setting aside fun activities in order to start homework   _____
15. Needs many reminders to start chores   _____

                       TOTAL SCORE: _____

16. Trouble planning for big assignments (knowing what to do first, second, etc.?   _____
17. Difficulty setting priorities when has a lot of things to do   _____
18. Becomes overwhelmed by long-term projects or big assignments   _____

                       TOTAL SCORE: _____

19. Backpack and notebooks are disorganized   _____
20. Desk or workspace at home or school is a mess   _____
21. Trouble keeping bedroom or locker tidy   _____

                       TOTAL SCORE: _____

(cont.)

Item	Score
22. Has a hard time estimating how long it takes to do something (such as homework?	_____
23. Often doesn't finish homework at night; rushes to get it done in school before class	_____
24. Slow getting ready for things (e.g., appointments, school, changing classes?	_____

TOTAL SCORE: _____

25. If the first solution to a problem doesn't work, has trouble thinking of a different one	_____
26. Resists changes in plans or routines	_____
27. Has problems with open-ended homework assignments (e.g., doesn't know what to write about when given a creative writing assignment?	_____

TOTAL SCORE: _____

High School Students Only

28. Lacks effective study strategies	_____
29. Doesn't check work for mistakes even when the stakes are high	_____
30. Doesn't evaluate performance and change tactics in order to increase success	_____

TOTAL SCORE: _____

31. Can't seem to save up money for a desired object; problems delaying gratification	_____
32. Doesn't see the value in earning good grades to achieve a long-term goal	_____
33. Seems to live in the present	_____

TOTAL SCORE: _____

KEY

Items	Executive Skill	Items	Executive Skill
1–3	Response inhibition	4–6	Working memory
7–9	Emotional control	10–12	Sustained attention
13–15	Task initiation	16–18	Planning/prioritization
19–21	Organization	22–24	Time management
25–27	Flexibility	28–30	Metacognition
31–33	Goal-directed persistence		

Child's Executive Skills Strengths

_____

_____

_____

Child's Executive Skills Weaknesses

_____

_____

_____

Executive Skills Questionnaire for Students

Big problem	1
Moderate problem	2
Mild problem	3
Slight problem	4
No problem	5

Item   Score

1. I act on impulse. _____

2. I get in trouble for talking too much in class. _____

3. I say things without thinking. _____

           TOTAL SCORE: _____

4. I say, "I'll do it later" and then forget about it. _____

5. I forget homework assignments or forget to bring home needed materials. _____

6. I lose or misplace belongings such as coats, notebooks, sports equipment, etc. _____

           TOTAL SCORE: _____

7. I get annoyed when homework is too hard or confusing or takes too long to finish. _____

8. I have a short fuse; am easily frustrated. _____

9. I get upset easily when things don't go as planned. _____

           TOTAL SCORE: _____

10. I have difficulty paying attention and am easily distracted. _____

11. I run out of steam before finishing my homework. _____

12. I have problems sticking with chores until they are done. _____

           TOTAL SCORE: _____

13. I put off homework or chores until the last minute. _____

14. It's hard for me to put aside fun activities in order to start homework. _____

15. I need many reminders to start chores. _____

           TOTAL SCORE: _____

16. I have trouble planning for big assignments (knowing what to do first, second, etc.? _____

17. It's hard for me to set priorities when I have a lot of things to do. _____

18. I become overwhelmed by long-term projects or big assignments. _____

           TOTAL SCORE: _____

19. My backpack and notebooks are disorganized. _____

20. My desk or workspace at home is a mess. _____

21. I have trouble keeping bedroom tidy. _____

           TOTAL SCORE: _____

(cont.)

Item   Score

22. I have a hard time estimating how long it takes to do something (such as homework?   _____

23. I often don't finish homework at night and rush to get it done in school before class.   _____

24. I'm slow getting ready for things (e.g., school or appointments?   _____

                                                                              TOTAL SCORE: _____

25. If the first solution to a problem doesn't work, I have trouble thinking of a different one.   _____

26. It's hard for me to deal with changes in plans or routines.   _____

27. I have problems with open-ended homework assignments (e.g., doesn't know what
    to write about when given a creative writing assignment?   _____

                                                                              TOTAL SCORE: _____

High School Students Only

28. I don't have effective study strategies.   _____

29. I don't check my work for mistakes even when the stakes are high.   _____

30. I don't evaluate my performance and change tactics in order to increase success.   _____

                                                                              TOTAL SCORE: _____

31. I can't seem to save up money for a desired object.   _____

32. I don't see the value in earning good grades to achieve a long-term goal.   _____

33. If I should be studying and something fun comes up, it's hard for me
    to make myself study.   _____

                                                                              TOTAL SCORE: _____

KEY			
Items	**Executive Skill**	**Items**	**Executive Skill**
1–3	Response inhibition	4–6	Working memory
7–9	Emotional control	10–12	Sustained attention
13–15	Task initiation	16–18	Planning/prioritization
19–21	Organization	22–24	Time management
25–27	Flexibility	28–30	Metacognition
31–33	Goal-directed persistence		

Your Executive Skills Strengths   **Your Executive Skills Weaknesses**

_____   _____

_____   _____

_____   _____

Executive Skills: Planning Interventions

Student Name: ___   Date: ___

I. Data Sources—check all that apply

_____ Parent Interview	_____ Parent Checklists	_____ Classroom Observation
_____ Teacher Interview	_____ Teacher Checklists	_____ Work Samples
_____ Student Interview	_____ Student Checklists	_____ Formal Assessment

II. Areas of Need—fill in applicable sections

Response Inhibition (RI): The capacity to think before acting

Specific problem behaviors (e.g., talks out in class; interrupts; says things without thinking)

1.

2.

3.

Working Memory (WM): The ability to hold information in memory while performing complex tasks

Specific problem behaviors (e.g., forgets directions; leaves homework at home; can't do mental arithmetic)

1.

2.

3.

Emotional Control (EC): The ability to manage emotions in order to achieve goals, complete tasks, or control or direct behavior

Specific problem behaviors (e.g., "freezes" on tests; gets frustrated when makes mistakes; stops trying in the face of challenge)

1.

2.

3.

Sustained Attention (SA): The capacity to maintain attention to a situation or task in spite of distractibility, fatigue, or boredom

Specific problem behaviors (e.g., fails to complete classwork on time; stops work before finishing)

1.

2.

3.

(cont.)

Task Initiation (TI): The ability to begin projects without undue procrastination, in an efficient or timely fashion

Specific problem behaviors (e.g., needs cues to start work; puts off long-term assignments)

   1.

   2.

   3.

Planning/Prioritization (P): The ability to create a roadmap to reach a goal or to complete a task

Specific problem behaviors (e.g., doesn't know where to start an assignment; can't develop a timeline for long-term assignments)

   1.

   2.

   3.

Organization (O): The ability to create and maintain systems to keep track of information or materials

Specific problem behaviors (e.g., doesn't write down assignments; loses books or papers)

   1.

   2.

   3.

Time Management (TM): The capacity to estimate how much time one has, how to allocate it, and how to stay within time limits and deadlines

Specific problem behaviors (e.g., doesn't work efficiently; can't estimate how long it takes to do something)

   1.

   2.

   3.

Goal-Directed Persistence (GDP): The capacity to have a goal, follow through to the completion of the goal, and not be put off by or distracted by competing interests

Specific problem behaviors (e.g., doesn't see connection between homework and long-term goals; doesn't follow through to achieve stated goals)

   1.

   2.

   3.

(cont.)

Flexibility (F): The ability to revise plans in the face of obstacles, setbacks, new information, or mistakes; it relates to an adaptability to changing conditions

Specific problem behaviors (e.g., gets stuck on one problem-solving strategy; gets upset by unexpected changes to schedule or plans)

1.

2.

3.

Metacognition (M): The ability to stand back and take a bird's-eye view of oneself in a situation; the ability to self-monitor and self-evaluate

Specific problem behaviors (e.g., doesn't have effective study strategies; difficulty catching or correcting mistakes)

1.

2.

3.

III. Establish Goal Behavior—select specific skill to work on

GOAL BEHAVIOR 1

Target Executive Skill: _____

Specific Behavioral Objective: _____

_____

_____

IV. Design Intervention

What environmental supports or modifications will be provided to help reach the target goal?

(cont.)

What specific skills will be taught, who will teach skill, and what procedure will be used to teach the skill(s)?

Skill:

Who will teach skill:

Procedure:

Skill:

Who will teach skill:

Procedure:

What incentives will be used to help motivate the student to use/practice the skill(s)?

How Will the outcome be measured?

V. Evaluate Intervention

Review date: _____

Was the behavioral objective met?   Yes, completely: ____   Yes, partially: ____   No: ____

(cont.)

Assessment of efficacy of intervention components:

Environmental Supports/Modifications
Were they put in place?
Were they effective?
Do they need to be continued?
Plan for fading supports:
Skill Instruction
Was the instruction implemented?
What was the outcome?
Does the instruction need to be continued?
Plan for fading instruction:
Incentives
Were incentives used?
Were they effective?
Do they need to be continued?
Plan for fading incentives:

Date for next review: _____

Forms for Developing Behavior Plans/Incentive Systems

A. Incentive Planning Sheet

Problem Behavior

Goal

Possible Rewards

Daily   Weekly   Long Term

Possible Contingencies

(cont.)

B. Contract

Child agrees to: _____

_____

_____

_____

To help child reach goal, parents or teacher(s) will: _____

_____

_____

_____

Child will earn: _____

_____

_____

_____

If child fails to meet agreement, child will: _____

_____

_____

_____

Executive Skills Self-Management Checklist

Element	What does student participation look like?	Check if included in intervention
Selection of target behavior	Student helps identify what behavior problem needs to be addressed.	
Definition	Student involved in developing operational definition of the target behavior (e.g., "keep hands to self during circle time").	
Selection of primary reinforcers	Student is asked to identify possible reinforcers; helps create a reinforcement menu.	
Performance goal	Student helps set a reasonable goal for the target behavior (e.g., "Remember to raise my hand x% of the time").	
Instructional prompt	Student helps decide the best way to remember to prompt for the behavior (e.g., use of kitchen timer or random self-cuing for on-task behavior).	
Observation	Student is responsible for monitoring the target behavior.	
Recording	Ask student best way to record the presence or absence of the target behavior.	
Evaluation	Student is at least partially responsible for determining when the goal was met (may include a system for verifying accuracy).	
Administration of secondary reinforcers	Student gives him- or herself points or tokens for exhibiting target behavior.	
Administration of primary reinforcers	When the student has accumulated enough points or tokens, he or she chooses reward from reinforcement menu.	
Monitoring	Student is responsible for charting or graphing performance over time.	

Getting to Know You

Name: _____

1. How do you spend your spare time? Check (v) all that apply and draw a circle around your favorite three activities.

☐ with family   ☐ TV/DVDs ☐ reading ☐ theater/dance   ☐ part-time job

☐ with friends   ☐ alone   ☐ sports   ☐ Internet, IM   ☐ video/computer games

☐ outdoors   ☐ sleeping ☐ writing ☐ listening to music   ☐ volunteering

☐ arts, crafts, building things   ☐ playing an instrument ☐ extracurricular activities at school

☐ dirt biking/four-wheeling   ☐ OTHER: _____

2. What talents do you have? Check all that apply and provide an example if you can.

☐ Athletic: _____   ☐ Artistic: _____

☐ Musical: _____   ☐ Writing: _____

☐ Communication: _____   ☐ Leadership: _____

☐ Performing arts: _____   ☐ Technology: _____

☐ Mechanical skills: _____   ☐ Math/sciences: _____

☐ Cooking, sewing: _____   ☐ Interpersonal skills: _____

☐ OTHER: _____

3. What personal qualities do you have that you consider to be strengths? Check up to five.

☐ leadership   ☐ patience   ☐ creativity   ☐ sense of humor ☐ independence

☐ caring, empathy ☐ hard worker ☐ loyalty   ☐ imagination   ☐ dependability

☐ determination ☐ optimism   ☐ self-control ☐ coping skills   ☐ problem solving

☐ persistence   ☐ ambition   ☐ honesty   ☐ organization   ☐ courage

☐ competitiveness ☐ extraversion (outgoing)   ☐ working well with others

☐ OTHER: _____

4. What areas of skill or knowledge would you like to become an expert in? List *any* topic that interests you, even if it is something you don't usually learn about in school (e.g., skateboarding, video games, sports statistics, cheerleading, horseback riding).

(cont.)

5. How do you learn best? Check all that apply.

   a. Group size:

   ☐ alone   ☐ small group (2–4 people)

   ☐ medium group (5–7 people)   ☐ whole class

   b. Learning style:

   ☐ visual   ☐ hands on

   ☐ listening   ☐ memorizing

   ☐ discussion   ☐ activity/experiential learning

   ☐ apprenticeship   ☐ taking notes

   ☐ reading   ☐ thinking about what I've read or heard

   ☐ OTHER: _____

   c. What is your preferred study environment?

   ☐ library   ☐ study hall at school

   ☐ bedroom   ☐ other room in my house

   ☐ with friends   ☐ public place (e.g., coffee shop)

   ☐ resource room   ☐ OTHER: _____

6. What are your preferred classroom activities? Check all that apply.

   ☐ lecture   ☐ discussions   ☐ projects

   ☐ debates   ☐ group games   ☐ presentations

   ☐ reading   ☐ creative writing   ☐ worksheets

   ☐ labs/experiments   ☐ cooperative learning   ☐ brainstorming

   ☐ outdoor activities   ☐ field trips   ☐ learn, then teach others

   ☐ role playing   ☐ simulations   ☐ taking tests

   ☐ self-directed learning ☐ individual research   ☐ doing homework

   ☐ movies/DVDs   ☐ working on the computer   ☐ teacher-led instruction

   ☐ doodling   ☐ daydreaming   ☐ talking with friends

   ☐ OTHER: _____

Morning Routine Checklist

Task	Check When Done
Hang up coats/outerwear in appropriate place	
Get out homework and place on right upper corner of desk	
Sharpen pencils and gather other materials needed for the first class	
Check the blackboard for instructions	
Follow instructions	

End-of-Day Routine Checklists

End-of-Day Routine—Checklist 1

Materials needed	Packed in bag
Assignment book filled in	
Spelling workbook	
Reading book	
Reading folder	
Social studies book	
Social studies folder	
Science book	
Science folder	
Math book	
Math folder	
Other (permission slips, notices, etc.):	

Signed: _____ Date: _____

(cont.)

End-of-Day Routine—Checklist 2

Steps to Follow	Check When Done
Hand in any homework assignments completed	
Hand in any in-class assignments completed	
Return any materials borrowed from classmates or teacher	
Tidy up desk surface; check floor around desk	
Gather all necessary materials to go home 1—Books 2—Notebooks 3—Folders 4—Assignment book 5—Worksheets 6—Slips/notices for parents 7—Clothing (hat, mittens, coat) 8—Gym clothes 9—Other	
Place appropriate materials in backpack	
Ask myself, Am I forgetting anything?	

Daily Homework Planner

Date: _____

Subject/assignment	Do I have all the materials?	Do I need help?	How long do you think it will take?	Start time	Stop time	How long did it take?
	Yes ☐ No ☐	Yes ☐ No ☐				
	Yes ☐ No ☐	Yes ☐ No ☐				
	Yes ☐ No ☐	Yes ☐ No ☐				
	Yes ☐ No ☐	Yes ☐ No ☐				
	Yes ☐ No ☐	Yes ☐ No ☐				
	Yes ☐ No ☐	Yes ☐ No ☐				

Attention-Monitoring Checklist

Date: _____

Time: _____

Class activity: _____

Was I paying attention?	
YES	NO

Desk Cleaning Checklist

STEP 1: GATHER NECESSARY MATERIALS

Materials needed	Check all that apply
Wastebasket	
Empty file folders	
Three-ring binders	
Paper clips	
Stapler	
Manila envelopes	

STEP 2: FOLLOW DESK-CLEANING PROCEDURE

Procedure	Check when done
Empty out desk.	
Sort everything into two piles: *Save/Don't Save*.	
Throw *Don't Save* pile in wastebasket.	
Sort *Save* Pile into two piles: 1. School stuff (books, unfinished assignments, assignments that are completed but the teacher wants me to save, pens, pencils, etc.) 2. Home stuff (notices/slips to give Mom, assignments I want to save but don't have to keep for teacher, uneaten snacks, etc.)	
Put "home stuff" in backpack to go home (in folders or manila envelopes if necessary).	
Sort school stuff: one pile for incomplete homework assignments, one pile for each subject (not current homework), one extra pile for "other."	
Organize each subject pile following teacher instructions (e.g., placing materials by date in three-ring binders or folders).	
Decide what to do with the "other" pile.	
Put all school materials neatly back in desk.	

Writing Template for a Five-Paragraph Essay

Introductory Paragraph

Sentence 1 summarizes what your essay is about:

Sentence 2 focuses in on the main point you want to make:

Sentence 3 adds more detail or explains why the topic is important:

Body Paragraphs

Paragraph 1, topic sentence:

    Supporting detail 1:

    Supporting detail 2:

    Supporting detail 3:

Paragraph 2, topic sentence:

    Supporting detail 1:

    Supporting detail 2:

    Supporting detail 3:

(cont.)

Paragraph 3, topic sentence:

Supporting detail 1:

Supporting detail 2:

Supporting detail 3:

Concluding Paragraph

Restate the most important point from the paper you want to make (what the reader should go away understanding):

Long-Term Project-Planning Sheet

STEP 1: SELECT TOPIC

What are possible topics?	What I like about this choice:	What I don't like:
1.		
2.		
3.		
4.		
5.		

Final Topic Choice:

STEP 2: IDENTIFY NECESSARY MATERIALS

What materials or resources do you need?	Where will you get them?	When will you get them?
1.		
2.		
3.		
4.		
5.		

(cont.)

STEP 3: IDENTIFY PROJECT TASKS AND DUE DATES

What do you need to do? (List each step in order)	When will you do it?	Check off when done
Step 1:		
Step 2:		
Step 3:		
Step 4:		
Step 5:		
Step 6:		
Step 7:		
Step 8:		
Step 9:		
Step 10:		

Reminder List

Include here any additional tasks or details you need to keep in mind as you work on the project. Cross out or check off each one as it is taken care of.

1. _____
2. _____
3. _____
4. _____
5. _____
6. _____
7. _____
8. _____
9. _____
10. _____

Tools for Studying

A. Menu of Study Strategies

Check off the ones you will use.

__ 1. Reread text	__ 8. Make concept maps	__ 15. Create a "cheat sheet"
__ 2. Reread/organize notes	__ 9. Make lists/organize	__ 16. Study with friend
__ 3. Read/recite main points	__ 10. Take practice test	__ 17. Study with study group
__ 4. Outline text	__ 11. Quiz myself	__ 18. Study session with teacher
__ 5. Highlight text	__ 12. Have someone else quiz me	__ 19. Study with a parent
__ 6. Highlight notes	__ 13. Study flash cards	__ 20. Ask for help
__ 7. Use study guide	__ 14. Memorize/rehearse	__ 21. OTHER: _____

B. Study Plan

Date	Day	Which strategies will I use? (write #)	How much time for each strategy?
	4 days before test	1. 2. 3.	1. 2. 3.
	3 days before test	1. 2. 3.	1. 2. 3.
	2 days before test	1. 2. 3.	1. 2. 3.
	1 day before test	1. 2. 3.	1. 2. 3.

C. Posttest Evaluation

How did your studying work out? Answer the following questions:

1. What strategies worked best?

2. What strategies were not so helpful?

3. Did you spend enough time studying?   Yes   No

4. If no, what more should you have done?

5. What will you do differently the next time?

Organizing Notebooks/Homework

A. Setting Up a Notebook/Homework Management System

System element	What will you use?	Got it (✓)
Place for unfinished homework		
Place for completed assignments		
Place to keep materials for later filing		
Notebooks or binder(s) for each subject		
Other things you might need: 1. 2. 3. 4.		

B. Maintaining a Notebook/Homework Management System

Task	Monday	Tuesday	Wednesday	Thursday	Weekend
Clean out "to be filed" folder					
Go through notebooks and books for other loose papers and file them					
Place all assignments (both finished and unfinished) in appropriate places					

Note-Taking Template: Cornell Method

Date: _____ Class: _____

Lecture Topic: _____

Key terms and concepts	Running notes	Reflections, questions, links to personal experience

Hard Times Board

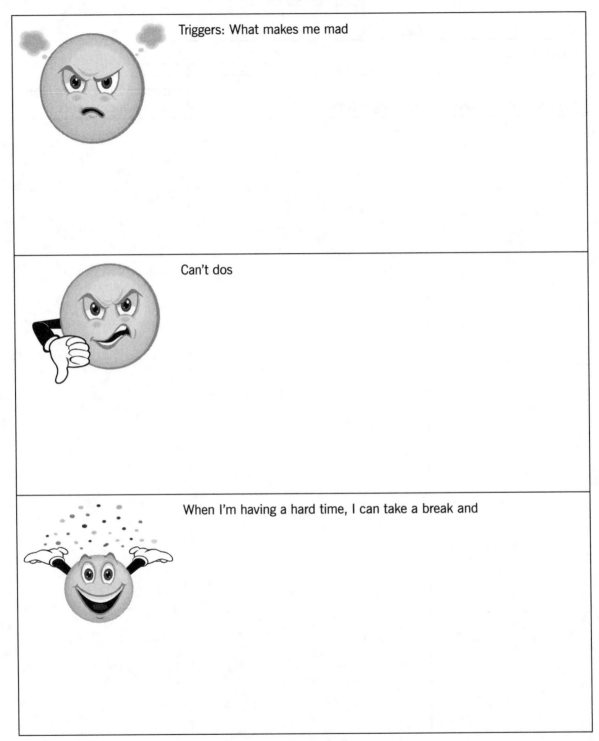

Triggers: What makes me mad

Can't dos

When I'm having a hard time, I can take a break and

Maintaining Self-Control

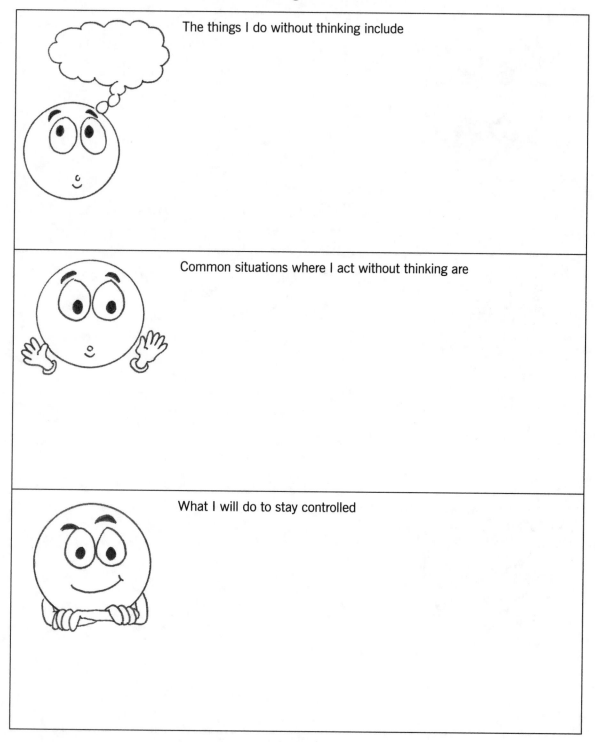

The things I do without thinking include

Common situations where I act without thinking are

What I will do to stay controlled

Worry Board

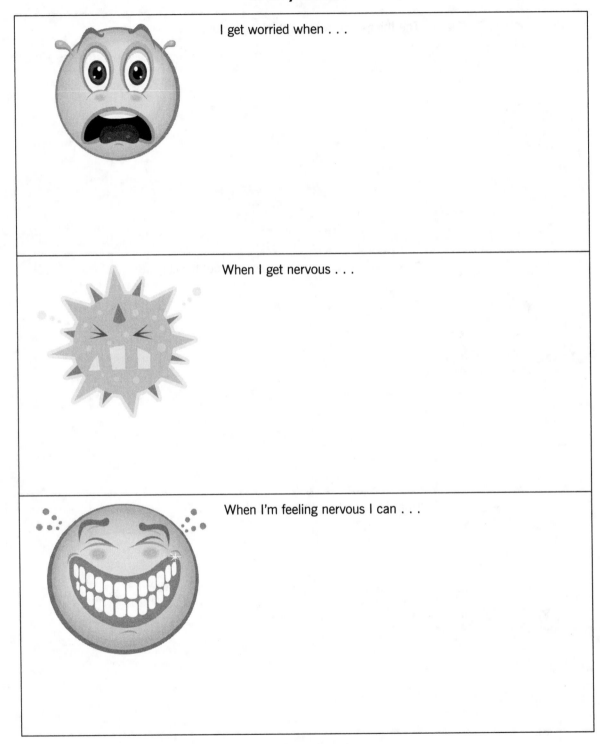

I get worried when . . .

When I get nervous . . .

When I'm feeling nervous I can . . .

Managing Changes in Plans or Schedules

A. Surprise! Card

Date: _____

Time	Activity
Surprise:	

B. Complaint Form

Date: _____

Nature of Complaint:

Why You Think the Situation Was Unfair:

What You Wish Had Happened:

Learning Not to Cry over Little Things

A. Upset Log

Date	Time	Duration of upset	Precipitating event

B. Contract

Here's what I can do instead of crying:

Here's what will happen if I can keep from crying when I'm upset:

Here's what will happen when I cry over little things:

Solving Problems Worksheet

What is the problem?
What are some possible things I (we) could do to solve the problem?
What will I (we) try first?
If this doesn't work, what can I (we) do?
How did it go? Did my (our) solution work?
What might I (we) do differently the next time?

Progress Monitoring: Response to Intervention

Student's Name: _____

Tier level	Intervention	Start date	Review date	Criterion for success	Measurement procedure	Outcome	Next step

References

Achenbach, T. M. (1991a). *Child Behavior Checklist.* Burlington, VT: University of Vermont.

Achenbach, T. M. (1991b). *Teacher Report Form.* Burlington, VT: University of Vermont.

Akshoomoff, N. (2005). The neuropsychology of autistic spectrum disorders. *Developmental neuropsychology, 27*(3), 307–310.

Alberto, P. A., & Troutman, A. C. (1999). *Applied behavior analysis for teachers* (5th ed.). Upper Saddler River, NJ: Prentice-Hall.

Anderson, V. (1998). Assessing executive functions in children: Biological, psychological, and developmental considerations. *Neuropsychological Rehabilitation, 8*(3), 319–349.

Anderson, V., Jacobs, P., & Anderson, P. (Eds.). (2008). *Executive functions and the frontal lobes: A lifespan perspective.* New York: Taylor & Francis.

Attwood, T. (2007). *The complete guide to Asperger's syndrome.* London: Jessica Kingsley.

Barkley, R. A. (1997). *ADHD and the nature of self-control.* New York: Guilford Press.

Batsche, G., Elliott, J., Graden, J. L., Grimes, J., Kovaleski, J. F., Prasse, D., Reschley, D. J., et al. (2005). *Response to intervention: Policy, considerations and implementation.* Alexandria, VA: National Association of State Directors of Special Education.

Briesch, A. M., & Chafouleas, S. M. (2009). Review and analysis of literature on self-management interventions to promote appropriate classroom behavior (1988–2008). *School Psychology Quarterly, 24,* 106–118.

Brown, T. E. (1996). *Brown Attention-Deficit Disorder Scales for Adolescents and Adults.* San Antonio, TX: Psychological Corporation.

Brown, T. E. (2001). *Brown Attention-Deficit Disorder Scales for Children and Adolescents.* San Antonio, TX: Psychological Corporation.

Buron, K. D., & Curtis, M. (2003). *The incredible 5–point scale.* Shawnee Mission, KS: Autism Asperger Publishing.

Conners, K. (2000). *Conners' Continuous Performance Test–II.* North Tonawanda, NY: Multi-Health Systems.

Dawson, P., & Guare, R. (1998). *Coaching the ADHD student.* North Tonowanda, NY: Multi-Health Systems.

Dawson, P., & Guare, R. (2009). *Smart but scattered: The revolutionary "executive skills" approach to helping children read.* New York: Guilford Press.

Delis, D., Kaplan, E., & Kramer, J. (2000). *Delis–Kaplan Executive Function Scale.* San Antonio, TX: Psychological Corporation.

DuPaul, G. J., Ervin, R. A., Hook, C. L., & McGoey, K. E. (1998). Peer tutoring for children with attention deficit hyperactivity disorder: Effects on classroom behavior and academic performance. *Journal of Applied Behavior Analysis, 31,* 579–592.

DuPaul, G. J., Power, T. J., Anastopoulos, A. D., & Reid, R. (1998). *ADHD Rating Scale-IV.* New York: Guilford Press.

Durston, S., Davidson, M. C., Mulder, M. J., Spicer, J. A., Galvan, A., Tottenham, N., et al. (2007). Neural and behavioral correlates of expectancy violations in attention-deficit hyperactivity disorder. *Journal of Child Psychology and Psychiatry, 48,* 881–889.

Fantuzzo, J. W., & Polite, K. (1990). School-based behavioral self-management: A review and analysis. *School Psychology Quarterly, 5,* 180–198.

Fantuzzo, J. W., Rohrbeck, C. A., & Azar, S. T. (1987). A component analysis of behavioral self-management interventions with elementary school students. *Child and Family Behavior Therapy, 9,* 33–43.

Gilotty, L., Kenworthy, L., Sirian, L., Black, D. O., & Wagner, A. E. (2002). Adaptive skills and executive function in autism spectrum disorders. *Child Neuropsychology, 8,* 241–248.

Gioia, G. A., Isquith, P. K., Guy, S. C., & Kenworthy, L. (2000). *Behavior Rating Inventory of Executive Function.* Odessa, FL: Psychological Assessment Resources.

Gresham, F. M., Restori, A. F., & Cook, C. R. (2008). To test or not to test: Issues pertaining to response to intervention and cognitive testing. *Communiqué, 37*(1), 5–7.

Guy, S. C., Isquith, P. A., & Gioia, G. A. (2004). *Behavior Rating Inventory of Executive Function: Self-report.* Odessa, FL: Psychological Assessment Resources.

Hackman, D., & Farah, M. (2009). Socioeconomic status and the developing brain, *Trends in Cognitive Sciences, 13,* 65–73.

Hallowell, E., & Ratey, J. (1994). *Driven to distraction.* New York: Pantheon.

Harris, K. R., Graham, S., Mason, L. H., & Friedlander, B. (2008). *Powerful writing strategies for all students.* Baltimore: Brookes.

Hart, T., & Jacobs, H. E. (1993). Rehabilitation and management of behavioral disturbances following frontal lobe injury. *Journal of Head Trauma Rehabilitation, 8,* 1–12.

Harvey V. S., & Chickie-Wolfe, L. (2007). *Fostering independent learning.* New York: Guilford Press.

Heaton, R. K. (1981). *Wisconsin Card Sorting Test (WCST).* Odessa, FL: Psychological Assessment Resources.

Huebner, D. (2006). *What to do when you worry too much.* Washington, DC: Magination Press.

Isquith, P. K., Crawford, J. S., Espy, K. A., & Gioia, G. A. (2005). Assessment of executive function in preschool-aged children. *Mental Retardation and Developmental Disabilities Research Reviews, 11,* 209–215.

Kagan, J. (1966). Reflection-impulsivity: The generality and dynamics of conceptual tempo. *Journal of Abnormal Psychology, 71,* 17–24.

Kolb, B., & Wishaw, Q. (1990). *Fundamentals of neuropsychology* (3rd ed.). New York: Freeman.

Korkman, M., Kirk, U., & Kemp, S. (2007). *NEPSY-II.* San Antonio, TX: Psychological Corporation.

Manly, T., Robertson, I. H., Anderson, V., & Nimmo-Smith, I. (1999). *The Test of Everyday Attention for Children (TEA-Ch).* Bury St. Edmunds, UK: Thames Valley Test Company.

Martin, C., Dawson, P., & Guare, R. (2007). *Smarts: Are we hardwired for success?* New York: AMACOM/American Management Association.

Merriman, D., & Codding, R. (2008). The effects of coaching on mathematics homework completion and accuracy of high school students with attention-deficit/hyperactivity disorder. *Journal of Behavioral Education, 17,* 339–355.

Mesulam, M.-M. (1985). *Principles of behavioral neurology.* Philadelphia: Davis.

Mitchum, K. J., Young, K. R., West, R. P., & Benyo, J. (2001). CWPASM: A classwide peer-assisted self-management program for general education classrooms. *Education and Treatment of Children, 24*(2), 111–140.

Mulhern, R. K., White, H. A., Glass, J. O., Kun, L. E., Leigh, L. Thompson, S. J., et al. (2004). Attentional functioning and white matter integrity among survivors of malignant brain tumors of childhood. *Journal of the International Neuropsychological Society, 10*(2), 180–189.

Nadebaum, C., Anderson, V., & Catroppa, C. (2007). Executive function outcomes following traumatic brain injury in young children: A five-year follow-up. *Developmental Neuropsychology, 32*(2), 703–728.

Naglieri, J., & Das, J. P. (1997). *Cognitive assessment system.* Itasca, IL: Riverside.

National Institute of Mental Health. (2001). *Teenage brain: A work in progress.* Available at *www.nimh.nih.gov/publicat/teenbrain.cfm.*

Neeper, R., Lahey, B. B., & Frick, P. A. (1990). *Comprehensive Behavior Rating Scale for Children.* San Antonio, TX: Psychological Corporation.

Noble, K., Norman, M., & Farah, M. (2005). Neurocognitive correlates of socioeconomic status in kindergarten children. *Developmental Science, 8,* 74–87.

Ozonoff, S., & Griffith, E. M. (2000). Neuropsychological function and the external validity of Asperger syndrome. In A. Klin, F. R. Volkmar, & S. S. Sparrow (Eds.), Asperger syndrome (pp. 72–96). New York: Guilford Press.

Paniagua, F. A. (1992). Verbal–nonverbal correspondence training with ADHD children. *Behavior Modification, 16,* 226–252.

Pelayo, R. P., Thorpy, M. J., & Glovinsky, P. (1988). Prevalence of delayed sleep phase syndrome among adolescents. *Sleep Research, 17,* 391.

Plessen, K., Bansal, R., Zhu, H., Whiteman, R., Amat, J., Quackenbush, G., et al. (2006). Hippocampus and amydala morphology in attention-deficit/hyperactivity disorder. *Archives of General Psychiatry, 63,* 795–807.

Pliszka, S. R. (2002). Neuroimaging and ADHD: Recent progress. *The ADHD Report, 10*(3), 1–6.

Pliszka, S., Glahn, D., Semrud-Clikeman, M., Franklin, C., Perez III, R., Xiong, J., et al. (2006). Neuroimaging of inhibitory control areas in children with attention deficit hyperactivity disorder who were treatment naive or in long-term treatment. *American Journal of Psychiatry, 163,* 1052–1060.

Plumer, P., & Stoner, G. (2005). The relative effects of classwide peer tutoring and peer coaching on the positive social behaviors of children with ADHD. *Journal of Attention Disorders, 9,* 290–300.

Porteus, S. D. (1959). *The Maze Test and clinical psychology.* Palo Alto, CA: Pacific Books.

Reitan, R. M., & Wolfson, D. (1985). *The Halstead–Reitan Neuropsychological Test Battery.* Tucson, AZ: Neuropsychological Press.

Schultz, B. K., Evans, S. W., & Serpell, Z. N. (2009). Preventing failure among middle school students with ADHD: A survival analysis. *School Psychology Review, 38*(1), 14–27.

Shaw, P., Eckstrand, K., Sharp, W., Blumenthal, J., Lerch, J., Greenstein, D., et al. (2007). Attention-deficit/hyperactivity disorder is characterized by a delay in cortical maturation. *Proceedings of the National Academy of Sciences, 104,* 19649–19654.

Sheslow, D., & Adams, W. (1990). *Wide Range Assessment of Memory and Learning.* Wilmington, DE: Wide Range.

Stallard, P. (2005). *A clinician's guide to think good–feel good.* Chichester, UK: Wiley.

Steege, M. W., & Watson, T. S. (2009). *Conducting school-based functional behavioral assessments* (2nd ed.): *A practitioner's guide.* New York: Guilford Press.

Tomlinson, C. A. (1999). *The differentiated classroom: Responding to the needs of all learners.* Alexandria, VA: Association for Supervision and Curriculum Development.

Tomlinson, C. A. (2001). *How to differentiate instruction in mixed-ability classrooms.* Alexandria, VA: Association for Supervision and Curriculum Development.

Vaquero, E., Gomez, C. M., Quintero, E. A., Gonzalez-Rosa, J. J., & Marquez, J. (2008). Differential prefrontal-like deficit in children after cerebellar astrocytoma and medulloblastoma tumor. *Behavioral and Brain Functions, 4,* 18.

Wechsler, D. (1991). *Wechsler Intelligence Scale for Children—Third Edition.* San Antonio, TX: Psychological Corporation.

Yeates, K., Swift, E., Taylor, H., Wade, S., Drotar, D., Stancin, E., et al. (2004). Short- and long-term outcomes following pediatric traumatic brain injury. *Journal of the International Neuropsychological Society, 10,* 412–426.

Ylvisaker, M., & Feeney, T. (2002). Executive functions, self-regulation, and learned optimism in pediatric rehabilitiation: A review and implications for intervention. *Pediatric Rehabilitation, 5*(2), 51–70.

Ylvisaker, M., & Feeney, T. (2008). Helping children without making them helpless: Facilitating development of executive self-regulation in children and adolescents. In V. Anderson, R. Jacobs, & P. Anderson (Eds.), *Executive functions and the frontal lobes: A lifespan perspective.* New York: Taylor & Francis.

Zimmerman, B. J., & Schunk, D. H. (2001). *Self-regulated learning and academic achievement.* Mahwah, NJ: Erlbaum.

Index

Page numbers followed by an *f* or *t* indicate figures or tables.